MW00624443

Congenital Heart Disease and Repair

Third Edition

By Allen D. Everett, M.D.
and D. Scott Lim, M.D.

Editorial Coordinator
Jasper Burns

Illustrated by
Paul Burns

Contributing Authors

Marcia L. Buck, Pharm.D.
David S. Cooper, M.D., M.P.H.
Jane E. Crosson, M.D.
Howard P. Gutgesell, M.D.
Jeffrey P. Jacobs, M.D.
Marshall L. Jacobs, M.D.
Stacie B. Peddy, M.D.
Luca A. Vricella, M.D.

13 digit ISBN: 978-0-9796252-4-4

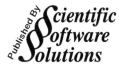

Published By *Scientific Software Solutions*

♻ Printed on recycled paper

Published by:

Scientific Software Solutions, Inc.
317 Monte Vista Avenue
Charlottesville, VA 22903
U.S.A.

Phone: 1.434.293.7661
Fax: 1.434.971.6528
Email: Info@PedHeart.com
Web: www.PedHeart.com, www.PedCath.com,
www.Congenital.org, www.HeartPassport.com

Dedications

To Martha Carpenter, MD and
Howard Gutgesell, MD, who taught me
what I know about Pediatric Cardiology
and being a Pediatric Cardiologist. – ADE

This book is dedicated to my children, Nyah
and Fanaye. By reading many bedtime stories, I
have become a better writer. – DSL

Publisher's Acknowledgments

Scientific Software would like to thank the authors for their diligence and cooperation in producing this important updated reference for congenital heart disease. In addition, Paul Burns deserves recognition for his superb illustrations. Jasper Burns designed, edited, and coordinated the development of the book. Emily Wilson, RN, BSN made an important contribution by proofing the manuscript. Logistical assistance was provided by Cara Shannon, who coordinated editorial meetings and supervised the final stages of production. Finally, Welton Gersony, MD Ziyad Hijazi, MD, John Kugler, MD, John Moore, MD, John Rhodes, MD, and Kas Sheehan, ARNP deserve special thanks for their time in reviewing the manuscript and for their valuable comments.

Preface to First Edition

The Illustrated Field Guide to Congenital Heart Disease and Repair was created to provide a pocket-sized visual resource for pediatric cardiologists to assist their discussions with staff, students, patients and their families.

This book is designed to serve a broad audience of medical students, residents and nurses. In addition, it is intended as a quick reference for anesthesiologists, general pediatricians and adult cardiologists who see only the occasional patient with congenital heart disease.

Our plan is to enlarge and improve this resource in future editions, with changes and additions that reflect user feedback and developments in the specialty. Already, a section on electrophysiology is in preparation.

We hope that our readers will favor us with comments and suggestions so that this book will become a truly valuable and convenient tool for the medical community.

Preface to Third Edition

The first two editions of the Field Guide have succeeded remarkably, with over 10,000 copies in print. As the field of pediatric cardiology has continued to evolve, so therefore must this Field Guide. To that end, we have revised every chapter as well as added new chapters on Hybrid Therapies and Percutaneous Valve Insertion. Additionally, the artwork of congenital heart disease has continued to evolve, with outstanding illustrations by Paul Burns.

We hope that the reader will continue to find the utility of this Field Guide in their daily work as well as educational endeavors.

Illustrated Field Guide to Congenital Heart Disease and Repair

Third Edition

THE AUTHORS

Allen D. Everett, MD
Associate Professor of Pediatrics
Johns Hopkins University
Helen B. Taussig Children's Heart Center
Baltimore, MD

D. Scott Lim, MD
Associate Professor of Pediatrics & Medicine
University of Virginia
Charlottesville, VA

Marcia L. Buck, PharmD
Associate Professor of Pediatrics
University of Virginia Children's Hospital
Charlottesville, VA

David S. Cooper, MD, MPH
Medical Director, Cardiovascular Intensive Care Unit and
   Extracorporeal Life Support Program
The Congenital Heart Institute of Florida (CHIF)
All Children's Hospital
Clinical Assistant Professor of Pediatrics
University of South Florida (USF)
St. Petersburg, FL

Jane E. Crosson, MD
Assistant Professor of Pediatrics
Pediatric Cardiology
Johns Hopkins School of Medicine
Baltimore, MD

Howard P. Gutgesell, MD
Professor of Pediatrics, Emeritus
University of Virginia
Virginia Children's Heart Center
Charlottesville, VA

Jeffrey P. Jacobs, MD, FACS, FACC, FCCP
Surgical Director of Heart Transplantation and
    Extracorporeal Life Support Programs
The Congenital Heart Institute of Florida (CHIF)
All Children's Hospital
Clinical Professor
Department of Surgery
University of South Florida (USF)
St. Petersburg, FL

Marshall L. Jacobs, MD
Center for Pediatric and Congenital Heart Diseases
Cleveland Clinic
Cleveland, OH

Stacie B. Peddy, MD
Director of Simulation, Cardiac Intensive Care Unit
Staff Cardiac Intensivist
Assistant Professor - Anesthesiology and Critical Care
    Medicine
Associate Fellowship Director - Pediatric Critical Care
The Children's Hospital of Philadelphia
Philadelphia, PA

Luca A. Vricella, MD, FACS
Associate Professor of Surgery and Pediatrics
Director, Pediatric Cardiac Surgery and Heart
    Transplantation
Johns Hopkins University
Baltimore, MD

Contents

Chapter 5. **Percutaneous Valve Insertion and Repair** - 205

Chapter 6. **Hybrid Therapies** - 215

Chapter 7. **Congenital Heart Surgeries** - 223

Chapter 8. Cardiac ICU Topics - 307

14

Chapter 9. **Introduction to Electrophysiology** - 339

Chapter 10. **Common Cardiac Pharmaceuticals** - 367

CHAPTER I. **THE NORMAL AND FETAL HEART**

By D. Scott Lim, MD and Allen D. Everett, MD

ANATOMY AND CIRCULATION

The systemic venous return to the heart is via the superior and inferior vena cava, which connect to the superior and inferior portions of the right atrium. The right atrium also receives flow of desaturated blood from the coronary sinus. Within the body of the right atrium is the Eustachian valve, which directs flow from the inferior vena cava across the foramen ovale. The right atrium connects to the right ventricle via the trileaflet tricuspid valve. The tricuspid valve has attachments to the right ventricular septum as well as free wall.

The right ventricle is a coarsely trabeculated pumping chamber, which becomes more smooth-walled as it transitions to the pulmonary outflow/subpulmonary valve area. The pulmonary valve is a trileaflet semilunar valve that sits to the left and anterior of the aortic valve. The main pulmonary artery branches into right and left pulmonary arteries, which connect to respective lung hila. Four or five pulmonary veins return oxygenated blood from the lung hila to the posterior right and left portions of the left atrium. The left atrium also contains a finger-like left atrial appendage, as opposed to the broader triangular right atrial appendage. The two atria are separated by the atrial septum, which consists of a thicker septum secundum and thinner septum primum.

The left atrium is connected to the left ventricle via the bileaflet mitral valve, which, unlike the tricuspid valve, does not have chordal attachments to the ventricular septum. The left ventricle is a smoothly trabeculated pumping chamber with mitral-aortic fibrous continuity. The aortic valve sits posterior and rightward of the pulmonary valve. The root of the aorta contains three cusps — the right coronary cusp gives rise to the right coronary artery, which courses around the base of the heart. The left coronary cusp gives rise to the left main coronary artery, which divides into the left anterior descending coronary and the circumflex coronary.

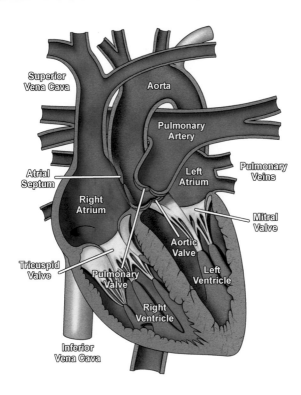

Internal Normal Heart
(Frontal View)

19

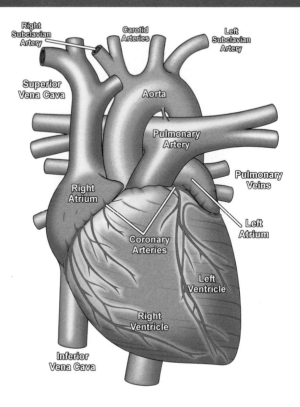

Above: External Normal Heart - Frontal View

Opposite:

> **Top - Internal Normal Heart**
>   Basal View from above
>
> **Bottom - External Normal Heart**
>   showing Coronary Artery Branches

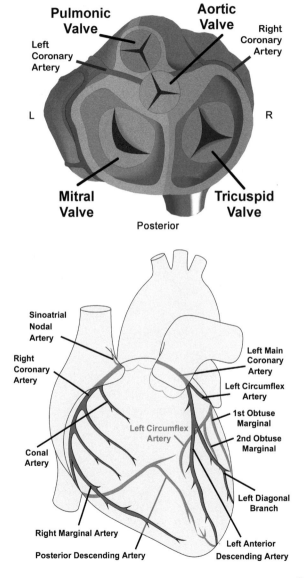

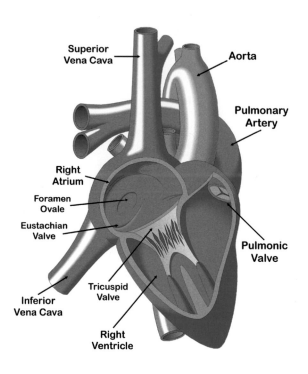

Internal Normal Heart
View from Right Side

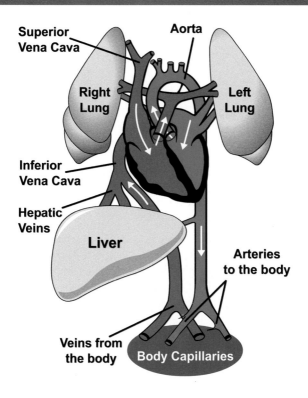

Superior Vena Cava

Aorta

Right Lung

Left Lung

Inferior Vena Cava

Hepatic Veins

Liver

Arteries to the body

Veins from the body

Body Capillaries

Normal Post-Natal Circulation

FETAL CIRCULATION

The unique aspect of the fetal cardiovascular circulation is its interface with the placenta.

ANTENATAL CIRCULATION – see diagrams **opposite**

Oxygenated blood (shown in red) enters the fetal circulatory system via placental transfer. Via the ductus venosus, the umbilical vein brings oxygenated blood to the inferior vena cava and right atrium, where it is directed by the Eustachian valve across the patent foramen ovale and into the left atrium. This allows the left ventricle to pump the most oxygenated blood to the coronary and carotid arteries.

Deoxygenated blood returning via the superior vena cava is preferentially directed across the tricuspid valve and into the right ventricle. The right ventricle pumps this blood into the pulmonary arteries, and across the patent ductus arteriosus into the descending aorta.

Antenatally, the lung is a relatively high resistance circuit, and therefore a smaller amount of blood flows through the pulmonary arteries and veins. The flow of blood is shown by the arrows. In the diagram **opposite**, top, oxygen-poor blood is shown in blue and moderately oxygenated blood in purple.

SHUNTS IN FETAL CIRCULATION

There are four unique structures in the fetal circulatory system through which blood is shunted (see the top diagram, **opposite**). These are the placenta, ductus venosus, foramen ovale; and ductus arteriosus.

Opposite:

> **Top** - Shunts in Fetal Circulation
> > 1 - Placenta; 2 - Ductus Venosus;
> > 3 - Foramen Ovale; 4 - Ductus Arteriosus
>
> **Bottom** - Circulation of oxygenated (red) and
> > deoxygenated (blue) blood through the fetal heart

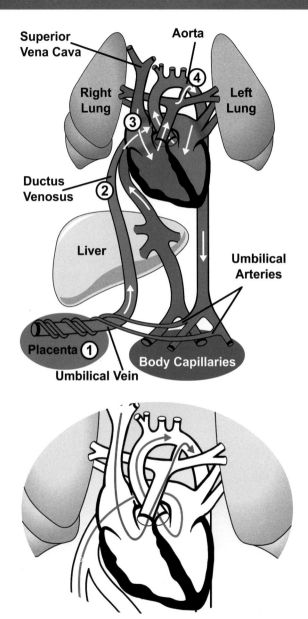

Superior
Vena Cava

Aorta

④

Right
Lung

Left
Lung

③

Ductus
Venosus

②

Liver

Umbilical
Arteries

Placenta ①

Body Capillaries

Umbilical Vein

25

THE FORAMEN OVALE

The foramen ovale is formed by a flap of septum primum that is pushed open by the flow of blood from the right to left atrium. Oxygenated blood from the ductus venosus is directed by the Eustachian valve toward the foramen ovale, and into the left heart. This shunts the blood with the highest oxygen content to the left heart for perfusion of the coronary arteries and brain. From the left atrium, the oxygenated blood is pumped into the left ventricle and into the aorta, which carries it to the body. From there it returns to the placenta via the umbilical arteries.

THE DUCTUS ARTERIOSUS

The ductus arteriosus connects the pulmonary artery to the aorta. This ductus shunts deoxygenated caval blood from the right ventricle to the descending aorta, bypassing the nonaerated lungs.

THE DUCTUS VENOSUS

The ductus venosus shunts oxygenated blood from the umbilical vein to the inferior vena cava, bypassing the sinusoids of the liver.

Opposite:

> **Top** - Foramen Ovale

> **Middle** - Ductus Arteriosus

> **Bottom** - Ductus Venosus

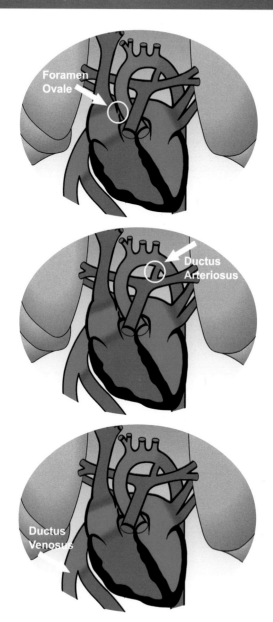

POSTNATAL CHANGES

At birth, the lungs inflate, decreasing pulmonary vascular resistance augmenting right ventricle blood flow. The resultant increase in pulmonary blood flow leads to an elevation in left atrial pressure, causing the septum primum flap to seal against the foramen ovale, and effectively separating the two atria. This also increases blood flow to the lungs, as blood entering the right atrium can no longer bypass the right ventricle and is now pumped through the pulmonary artery into the lungs.

In response to the increased oxygenation of the blood, the surrounding smooth muscle of the ductus arteriosus permanently constricts, eliminating ductal blood flow. Similarly, the ductus venosus closes off soon after birth.

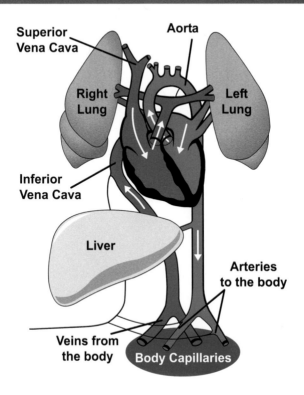

Normal Post-Natal Circulation

CHAPTER 2. **CONGENITAL HEART DEFECTS**

By Allen D. Everett, MD and D. Scott Lim, MD

Anatomic Description
In this rare defect, the pulmonary valve tissue is poorly-formed and there is significant insufficiency. This frequently results in massive dilatation of the pulmonary arteries, which may lead to extrinsic compression of the bronchial airway and abnormal development of the ventilatory tree. There can also be an associated ventricular septal defect (VSD). This defect is also referred to sometimes as tetralogy of Fallot (see page 92) with absent pulmonary valve because the VSD can be a malalignment type (see page 116).

Pathophysiology
There can be significant variability in the degree of bronchial compression secondary to distal pulmonary artery dilatation. In significant cases, there is marked respiratory impairment. In the presence of a ventricular septal defect, right to left shunting can occur leading to systemic desaturation, which may be worsened by associated airway obstruction.

Therapy
Plication of the pulmonary arteries, pulmonary valve replacement[1] and closure of the VSD[2] are the goals of surgical therapy in severe cases. Less severe cases may only require VSD closure. Most attempts at palliating severe cases of associated bronchial compression have been disappointing.

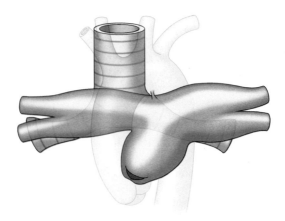

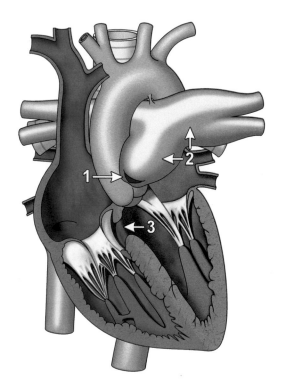

Above: Absent pulmonary valve

1. Absent or insufficient pulmonary valve
2. Dilatation of the pulmonary arteries
3. Ventricular septal defect (VSD)

Opposite: Note enlarged pulmonary arteries and obstructed bronchial tree.

---

[1] See page 226 for surgical replacement of the pulmonary valve.

[2] See page 302 for surgical repair of the ventricular septal defect.

Anatomic description

This is an uncommon defect, in which the left coronary artery is abnormal in either origin or course.

In the normal heart, the left coronary artery arises from the left aortic sinus. However, the left coronary artery can originate from the pulmonary artery (as shown in the illustration **opposite** and at the top on page 37), from the right aortic sinus (see the middle and bottom pictures on page 37), or as separate ostia for the anterior descending and circumflex branches. When arising from the right aortic sinus, the left coronary can course either posterior to the aorta, in between the aorta and pulmonary artery, in the interventricular septum, or anterior to the pulmonary artery. When the coronary artery courses between the aorta and pulmonary artery, its ostia is frequently slit-like and stenotic.

Pathophysiology

In patients with pulmonary arterial origin of the left coronary artery, the left ventricular myocardium is inadequately perfused with deoxygenated pulmonary arterial blood at a lower driving pressure, leading to ischemia and a dilated cardiomyopathy. Myocardial perfusion may be further compromised by collateral formation from the higher pressure right to the lower pressure left coronary system, stealing flow from the myocardium and shunting it to the pulmonary artery.

In patients with right aortic sinus origin of the left coronary artery or left coronary sinus origin of the right coronary, the anomalous vessel may course between aorta and pulmonary artery and dynamic compression can occur (see page 37, middle). This subtype of anomalous left coronary artery can be associated with exercise-induced chest pain and sudden cardiac death. Passage of the left coronary artery anterior to the pulmonary valve is a risk factor for tetralogy of Fallot repair.[1]

---

[1]See page 294 for tetralogy of Fallot repair.

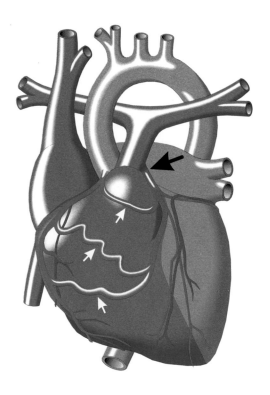

Above: Anomalous left coronary artery

Left coronary artery (black arrow) arises from pulmonary artery. Collateral coronary arteries are indicated by white arrows.

Therapy

Currently, for pulmonary artery origin, surgical ligation at the pulmonary side, reimplantation[1] or, historically, tunneling of the LCA to the aorta is performed (see Takeuchi Procedure[2]). Surgical repair should be considered even in the presence of severe cardiomyopathy. For anomalous origin of the RCA or LCA, the vessel can either be tunneled or reimplanted, or it can be bypassed with a mammary graft.

Below: Normal Heart (from above)

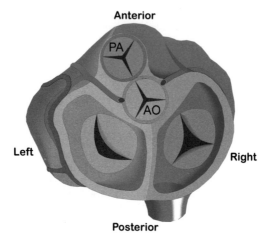

Opposite:

> **Top** - Left coronary artery arises from the pulmonary artery.
> **Middle** - Left coronary artery arises from the right aortic sinus and passes between aorta and pulmonary artery.
> **Bottom** - Left coronary artery arises from the right aortic sinus and passes anterior to the pulmonary artery.
>
> LCA – left coronary artery,
> RCA – right coronary artery

---

[1] See page 228 for surgical reimplantation.

[2] See page 292 for Takeuchi Procedure.

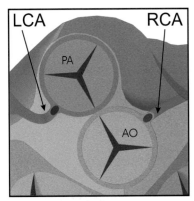

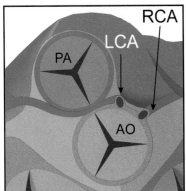

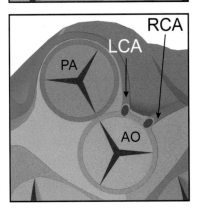

Anatomic Description

In this defect at least one but not all pulmonary veins connect anomalously to the right heart. Frequently this involves the right pulmonary veins draining to the right heart by way of the superior or inferior venae cavae. There are many variations of this anomaly, but the most common is right upper pulmonary vein draining into the superior vena cava. This defect can occur in association with an ASD and lung abnoralities (scimitar syndrome).

Pathophysiology

Patients with this defect are usually asymptomatic and may be identified serendipitously. The draining of pulmonary veins to the right atrium is physiologically identical to that of an atrial septal defect (i.e. right atrial and ventricular volume overload, with chamber dilation). The greater the number of veins draining anomalously, the larger the shunt. A significant shunt (Qp:Qs > 1.5:1) will result in right atrial and ventricular dilation and is an indication for surgical repair.

Therapy

The surgical repair of Partial Anomalous Pulmonary Venous Return involves redirecting the anomalous pulmonary veins to the left atrium. If dealing with left pulmonary veins that drain superiorly to the innominate vein, they may be directly re-anastomosed to the left atrial appendage. If dealing with anomalous right pulmonary veins draining to the superior vena cava, they may be tunneled through the atrial septal defect to the left atrium.[1]

Opposite: (Top) - In this example, the anomalous right upper pulmonary veins (RUPV and RMPV) enter the superior vena cava (SVC); (**Bottom**) - In this example, the anomalous left upper pulmonary vein enters the superior vena cava by way of the innominate vein.

(RLPV - right lower pulmonary vein, RMPV - right middle pulmonary vein, RUPV - right upper pulmonary, LUPV - left upper pulmonary vein, LLPV - left lower pulmonary vein, SVC – superior vena cava)

---

[1] See page 230 for this type of surgical repair of Partial Anomalous Pulmonary Venous Return.

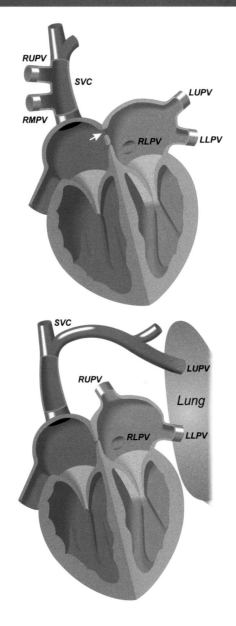

Anatomic Description

In this defect, all the pulmonary veins are abnormal with re-spect to how they connect to the heart.

There are various forms of this defect, but all involve the oxygenated blood from the lungs being carried by the pul-monary veins back to the right side of the heart rather than to the left atrium. Therefore, systemic blood flow requires right-to-left shunting across an associated atrial septal defect.

In the most common form of this defect (shown in the illus-tration, **opposite**), the pulmonary veins meet in a confluence behind the left atrium and connect to the innominate vein by a "vertical vein". The innominate vein then carries the mix of pulmonary venous and systemic venous blood to the right superior vena cava and, in turn, right atrium. This is known as the supracardiac type.

Less commonly, the pulmonary venous confluence may drain below the diaphragm and connect to the portal venous system for return to the right atrium (infracardiac – upper illustration on page 43). This type of anomalous pulmonary venous re-turn is always associated with obstruction to pulmonary ve-nous return.

Another type is with the pulmonary veins returning to the coronary sinus, which drains to the right atrium (intracardiac – lower illustration on page 43). It is also possible for the veins to be of mixed type. For example, the left sided veins may return via a supracardiac route and the right-sided veins via an infracardiac route.

Occasionally, there can also be associated pulmonary vein stenosis.

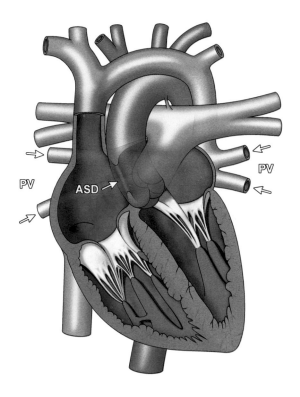

Above: Supracardiac Anomalous Pulmonary Venous connection to the superior vena cava

ASD - atrial septal defect, PV - pulmonary veins

Pathophysiology

Children with total anomalous pulmonary venous return present with varying degrees of cyanosis. If there is no obstruction to blood flow, infants and children with this defect have obligate mixing of saturated and desaturated blood in the right atrium, and right-to-left shunting of partially deoxygenated blood across the atrial septal defect. However, if there is obstruction to pulmonary venous return, there may be severe cyanosis with rapid development of acidosis.

The degree of obstruction to pulmonary venous return may be mild with the supracardiac type, as there may be mild compression of the vertical vein between the left pulmonary artery and left bronchus. However, in infracardiac drainage, the anomalous pulmonary veins are always obstructed and require immediate surgical repair. Obstructed pulmonary venous return is a surgical emergency.

Therapy

Surgical treatment of Total Anomalous Pulmonary Venous Return involves creating an anastamosis between the pulmonary venous confluence and the left atrium.[1] The anomalous connection (vertical vein or infracardiac vein) should then be ligated to prevent left-to-right shunting, and the atrial septal defect should be closed.

Opposite: Varieties of Anomalous Pulmonary Venous Return

> **Top – Infracardiac type:** Anomalous pulmonary venous connection to the inferior vena cava via the portal circulation

> **Bottom – Intracardiac type:** Anomalous pulmonary venous connection to the right atrium (see arrow), often at the coronary sinus

> (PV - pulmonary veins, HPV – hepatic portal vein)

---

[1] See page 232 for surgical treatment of Total Anomalous Pulmonary Venous Return.

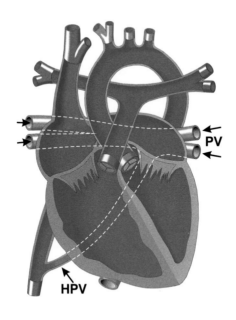

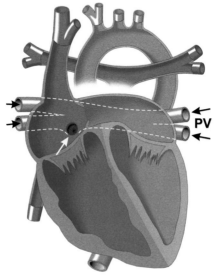

43

Anatomic Description

In valvar aortic stenosis, the leaflets may be thickened, or bi-cuspid and rarely unicuspid. There can be associated defects such as patent ductus arteriosus, subaortic stenosis, mitral stenosis, or coarctation of the aorta. With more than mild stenosis, compensatory left ventricular hypertrophy is present. Less frequently, the obstruction does not involve the aortic valve itself but consists of narrowing of the proximal aortic lumen above the valve (supravalvar stenosis) or of the left ventricular outflow tract (subvalvar stenosis). Supravalvar aortic stenosis can be associated with coronary artery osteal obstruction. Subvalvular aortic stenosis can lead to insufficiency of the aortic valve.

Pathophysiology

The natural history of aortic valvular stenosis is progressive, albeit slowly in most cases. This results in increasing after-load on the left ventricle, resultant hypertrophy, increased myocardial oxygen demand, and subendocardial ischemia. Because ventricular arrhythmia and sudden cardiac death can occur rarely in severe cases, exercise limitations have been recommended.

Therapy

For patients with severe obstruction due to valvular aortic stenosis (peak-to-peak gradient > 70mmHg or > 50mmHg with symptoms), intervention is warranted to decrease the risk of sudden death. Balloon valvuloplasty[1] is usually the initial palliative procedure, even in neonates, but most patients will ultimately require valve replacement. Surgical possibilities include the Ross Procedure[2], or valve replacement with biologic or mechanical valves. Research trials on percutaneous aortic valve replacement are in progress.

For patients with severe supravalvar stenosis, surgical aortoplasty may be performed. Patients with less severe degrees of subvalvar aortic stenosis are often referred for surgical resection because of the risk of aortic insufficiency. In cases of severe subvalvular obstruction, the Konno procedure[3] may be performed, often in combination with the Ross repair or mechanical valve replacement.

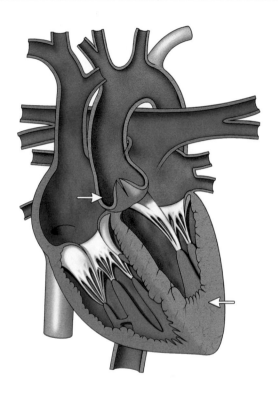

Above: Valvar aortic stenosis (upper arrow) with left ventricular hypertrophy (lower arrow)

---

[1] See page 188 for balloon valvuloplasty.

[2] See page 286 for the Ross Procedure.

[3] See page 268 for the Konno Procedure.

Anatomic Description

Aortopulmonary Window is a rare congenital heart defect in which there is a connection (window) between the aorta and the main or right pulmonary artery. Aortopulmonary window can occur as an isolated defect, or in association with an interrupted aortic arch.

Pathophysiology

An aortopulmonary window results in a left-to-right shunt, with pulmonary overcirculation and left heart dilatation. With large defects, pulmonary hypertension can be present.

Therapy

Surgical treatment of this defect is the mainstay of therapy and must be performed early to prevent irreversible pulmonary hypertension.[1]

Below: The dotted areas indicate the portions of the pulmonary artery in which communications with the aorta may occur.

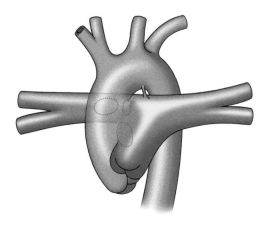

---

[1] See page 234 for surgical treatment of Aortopulmonary Window.

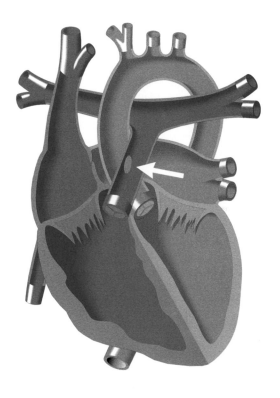

Above: Aortopulmonary window, indicated by arrow

Anatomic Description

Atrial Septal Defects (ASD) most commonly occur as defects in septum primum within the fossa ovalis (secundum atrial septal defects). Less commonly, the defect can involve septum secundum near the superior vena cava (sinus venosus atrial septal defects), or the coronary sinus. For defects in the primum septum near the atrioventricular valves, see atrioventricular septal defect, partial (see page 52).

Pathophysiology

As the right heart is quite compliant, there is a left-to-right shunt through the atrial septal defect. With time in larger defects, this results in right atrial and ventricular dilatation. Over time, right atrial fibrosis can occur and act as substrate for late-occurring atrial arrhythmias. With right ventricular dilatation, tricuspid annular dilatation can occur, resulting in tricuspid insufficiency. With large shunts, pulmonary congestion occurs, and uncommonly, pulmonary hypertensive changes can complicate the course. With severe pulmonary hypertension in older unoperated patients, right-to-left shunting and cyanosis can occur. The opportunity for right-to-left shunting creates a risk for systemic emboli and stroke.

Therapy

Small shunts that do not cause enlargement of the right heart chambers (Qp:Qs < 1.5:1) do not require therapy. The previous mainstay of therapy has been surgical closure, either by direct suture anastamosis or patch closure, using autologous pericardium or synthetic material.[1] Currently, for the majority of secundum atrial septal defects, transcatheter device therapy has become the treatment of choice.[2]

Opposite, bottom:

Arrow shows direction of blood flow through the ASD - from left atrium to right atrium. Blood flow continues through the tricuspid valve into the right ventricle. (Pulmonary artery and aorta removed for clarity.)

---

[1] See page 238 for patch closure of ASD.

[2] See page 172*ff* for transcatheter closure of ASD.

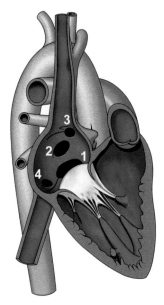

Above: Types of ASD viewed from the right atrium
1. Primum; 2. Secundum; 3. Superior Sinus Venosus;
4. Inferior Sinus Venosus

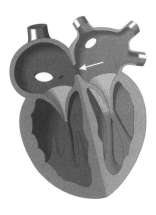

Anatomic Description

Atrioventricular Septal Defect (AVSD, also called Endocardial Cushion Defect or Atrioventricular Canal Abnormality) is due to incomplete fusion of the endocardial cushions, which give rise to the primum atrial septum, atrioventricular valves, and inlet portion of the ventricular septum. Therefore, the spectrum of this defect involves malformation of the mitral and tricuspid valves, resulting in a common atrioventricular valve that straddles the ventricular septum. There can be varying degrees of associated atrial (primum defect) or ventricular septal defects (inlet type). The common valve can be committed more to the right or left ventricle, leading to underdevelopment of the contralateral ventricle. AVSD can also exist in combination with Tetralogy of Fallot (see page 92), Double Outlet Right Ventricle (see page 64), and Subaortic Stenosis (see page 44). AVSD is very common in children with trisomy 21, but is also seen in non-trisomic patients.

Pathophysiology

There can be a significant left-to-right shunt at atrial and ventricular levels, leading to pulmonary over-circulation and congestive heart failure. Variable degrees of atrioventricular valve regurgitation can complicate this lesion. Neonates often have persistently elevated pulmonary vascular resistance and may not be symptomatic. The electrocardiogram is diagnostic with a leftward, superior axis, having a counterclockwise frontal plane vector loop.

Therapy

This defect almost invariably requires surgical intervention, with the optimal timing between 4 and 6 months of life.[1]

Opposite:

>   **Top** - Front view of heart showing atrial component (primum ASD) and ventricular component (inlet VSD)

>   **Bottom** – View of the heart from above showing single valvular opening (common atrioventricular valve) in blue

---

[1] See page 242 for surgical repair of AVSD - Complete.

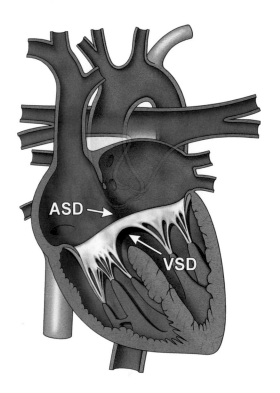

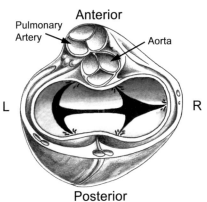

Anatomic Description

This defect is a less severe form of the complete atrioventricular septal defect, consisting of:

1. A defect in the primum portion of the atrial septum (primum atrial septal defect)

2. A malformation of the mitral valve (a cleft in the anterior leaflet of the valve)

Unlike the complete atrioventricular septal defect, there are always two separate atrioventricular valves (mitral and tricuspid) and the ventricular septum is intact.

Pathophysiology

The effect of this lesion is a left-to-right shunt at the atrial level, leading to right atrial and ventricular dilatation and pulmonary overcirculation. There can be varying degrees of mitral regurgitation from the cleft anterior leaflet. Mitral insufficiency can increase the degree of the left-to-right shunt and left atrial enlargement.

Therapy

Surgical repair, involving patch closure of the atrial septal defect and suturing of the mitral valve cleft, is the mainstay of treatment.[1]

Opposite:

Top: View of heart from left side showing:
1 - cleft in anterior leaflet of mitral valve
2 - atrial septal defect

Bottom: View of the heart from above showing:
1 - cleft in anterior leaflet of the mitral valve
2 - atrial septal defect

---

[1] See page 244 for surgical repair of AVSD-Partial.

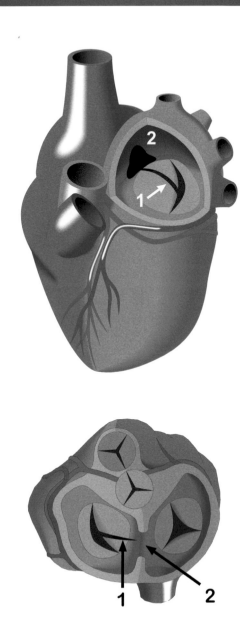

Coarctation of the Aorta

Anatomic Description

Coarctation of the Aorta is characterized by a narrowing of the lumen of the aorta. This may consist of a posterior shelf-like obstruction in the juxtaductal region or complete tubular hypoplasia of the aorta. With coarctation in the juxtaductal region, patency of the ductus arteriosus limits the degree of obstruction. Less commonly, aortic coarctation can occur in the transverse aortic arch, or rarely, in the abdominal aorta. Frequently, the aortic valve is bicuspid. Infrequently, coarctation can be part of a constellation of left sided obstructions (supravalvar mitral ring, subaortic stenosis). Uncommonly, coarctation of the aorta is associated with an aberrant right subclavian artery arising distal to the coarctation resulting in coarctation without the characteristic physical finding of right arm hypertension.

Pathophysiology

The obstruction to aortic blood flow caused by the coarctation leads to an increase in afterload on the left ventricle. There is a resultant higher blood pressure proximal to the obstruction, and lower blood pressure distal (usually leading to a limb systolic blood pressure discrepancy). In severe cases, distal organ perfusion can be compromised. Additionally, the severe increase in afterload after ductal closure can lead to left ventricular failure and pulmonary hypertension. In less severe cases, coarctation can present with long-standing upper body hypertension.

Therapy

When coarctation presents in infancy, palliation with prostaglandins to open or maintain ductal patency can be lifesaving. Surgery is the standard in infant coarctation, and has evolved over the years in an attempt to limit the late complications of recurrence or aneurysm formation.

Recently, resection of the coarctation and ductal tissue with an extended end-to-end anastomosis[1] has become a popular surgical approach. In the older patient with coarctation, both surgical and transcatheter approaches may be offered. Balloon angioplasty[2] has met with moderate success in discrete coarctations, with a small but significant risk of late aneurysm formation. Transcatheter stent placement may provide similar success with reduced recurrence or aneurysm risk.[3]

54

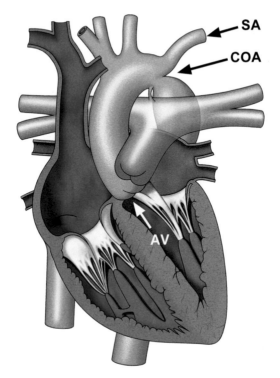

Above: Coarctation of the aorta

  COA - coarctation
  SA - subclavian artery
  AV - aortic valve

---

[1] See page 248 for the extended end-to-end anastomosis procedure.
[2] See page 196 for balloon angioplasty of coarctation.
[3] See page 200 for transcatheter stent placement.

Anatomic Description

In this rare defect, there is an abnormal communication between a coronary artery and an intracardiac chamber (atrial or
ventricular) or pulmonary artery.

Pathophysiology

Depending on the size of the communication, there can be
a significant left-to-right shunt, leading to volume overload
and chamber dilation. There also can be significant dilation
of the involved coronary artery proximal to where it enters
the receiving chamber. With a large shunt, perfusion of the
distal myocardium may be compromised because of prefer-
ential flow into the low resistance right heart structures.

Therapy

Most often, small coronary artery fistulae are asymptomatic
and thought to need no intervention. Large coronary artery
fistulae may be closed surgically or occluded with a coil or
occlusion device introduced through a catheterization procedure. The surgical procedure involves closing the fistula with
sutures on the surface of the heart chamber it enters, though
there are several other approaches that may be used.

Opposite:

>   **Top** - Circle shows point of entry into the heart
>   chamber (right ventricle)

>   **Bottom** - View from above of heart with dilated left
>   coronary artery (LCA) because of increased flow
>   secondary to a LCA fistula.

>   LCA – left coronary artery
>   RCA – right coronary artery
>   AO – aorta
>   PA – pulmonary artery

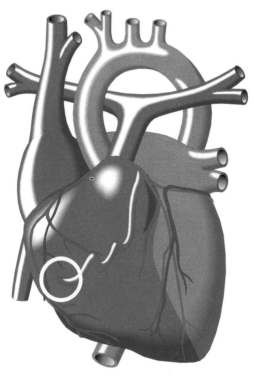

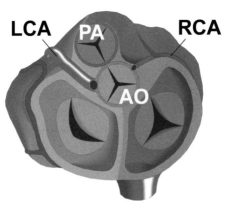

Dextrocardia

Anatomic Description
The term Dextrocardia is reserved for when the heart is in the right chest with its apex pointing to the right. In contrast, the term dextro-position refers to the heart in the right chest, but with the apex pointing to the left (possibly occurring secondary to right lung hypoplasia).

Dextrocardia is often associated with a myriad of other anomalies of situs.

Pathophysiology
Isolated Dextrocardia imposes no hemodynamic burden on the circulatory system. However, associated anomalies of situs or related cardiac defects can have a significant effect.

Therapy
Isolated Dextrocardia requires no therapy. However, if associated with abdominal visceral situs abnormalities (asplenia or polysplenia), intestinal malrotation must be evaluated and treated surgically. Antibiotic prophylaxis in asplenic patients must be instituted in infancy.

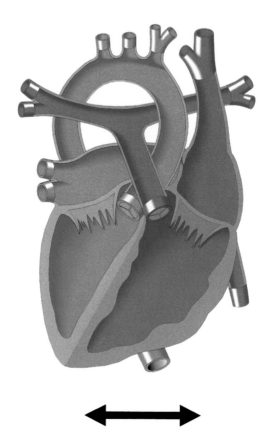

Above: Dextrocardia - Mirror Image of Normal Heart
  (frontal view)

Anatomic Description

Dilated Cardiomyopathy is the anatomic and functional result of either an intrinsic abnormality of the myocardium, or chronic injury to the myocardium. In the pediatric-age population, it is frequently suspected to be the end-result of occult viral myocarditis.

In order to maintain systolic function of the diseased myocardium, the ventricle dilates, leading to increased wall stress and compensatory hypertrophy. With significant ventricular dilation, the atrioventricular valve annulus can dilate, leading to valvar regurgitation. Due to myocardial dysfunction, elevated filling pressures, and atrioventricular valve insufficiency, the atria can become dilated.

Pathophysiology

The ability of the ventricle to contract is impaired, and cardiac output is decreased and partially compensated for by tachycardia. Due to diastolic dysfunction of the cardiomyopathic left ventricle, the left atrial filling pressures are elevated, which can be exacerbated by mitral insufficiency. In severe states, this leads to pulmonary venous congestion, pulmonary edema, and pulmonary hypertension. Atrial and ventricular stretch results in increased release of the cardiac hormone, B-type natriuretic peptide.

Therapy

Diuretics continue to be the mainstay of therapy. Recently, decreasing myocardial oxygen demand by beta-blocker therapy with carvedilol and angiotensin converting enzyme inhibitors (ACE) may be beneficial in pediatric heart failure patients. In end-stage heart failure in adult patients, ventricular assist devices have found utility, and may find a role in selected pediatric patients as a bridge to transplant or as destination therapy. Ultimately, cardiac transplantation remains a limited option for severely affected patients with dilated cardiomyopathy.

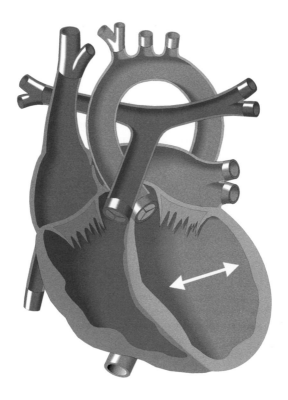

Above: Dilated cardiomyopathy

Anatomic Description

Double-chambered right ventricle is a rare form of congenital heart disease in which anomalous muscle bundles cause mid-cavitary obstruction within the right ventricle. The muscle bundles segregate the right ventricle into a high-pressure lower chamber, and a lower pressure outflow portion of the right ventricle.

Double-chambered right ventricle is frequently, but not uniformly associated with a perimembranous ventricular septal defect (see page 119). It is less commonly associated with sub-aortic obstruction, and rarely with hypertrophic cardiomyopathy.

Pathophysiology

Data from early and limited natural history studies indicate that double-chambered right ventricle tends to be progressive. The right ventricular outflow tract obstruction induces pressure overload on the right ventricle, with resultant right ventricular hypertrophy and in turn worsening obstruction from the anomalous muscle bundles. Right-sided heart failure has been reported in advanced cases, as well as right-to-left shunting at the atrial level and resultant cyanosis. Atrial and ventricular arrhythmias can also develop as a consequence of the hemodynamic burden.

Therapy

Medical therapy is not beneficial in treating isolated double-chambered right ventricle. Significant right ventricular hypertension, particularly when the right ventricular pressures approach or exceed systemic pressures, is an indication for surgical resection.

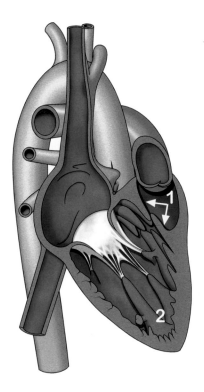

Above: Double-chambered right ventricle, shown from the right ventricle free wall side

1 - Muscle bundles in the RV outflow, indicated by arrows, and the low pressure portion of the RV

2 - The high pressure portion of the RV

Double-Inlet Left Ventricle

Anatomic Description
In most forms of this rare defect, ventricular inversion with ventricular-arterial discordance occurs (rarely, this lesion can occur in a D-looped heart). Both atrioventricular valves empty into the left ventricle, which is commonly connected to a rudimentary and hypoplastic right ventricle (bulboventricle) by a ventricular septal defect (bulboventricular foramen). The right ventricle can give rise to both great vessels (double-outlet right ventricle, see page 66) or the aorta alone (frequently associated with a stenotic pulmonary artery arising from the left ventricle). There may be an associated atrial septal defect and possible abnormalities of situs.

Pathophysiology
This defect results in complete intracardiac mixing of both systemic and pulmonary venous blood. The degree of systemic oxygenation is dependent upon the presence of pulmonary arterial obstruction. In the absence of pulmonary stenosis, these infants will have pulmonary over-circulation and congestion. In the presence of pulmonary stenosis, the circulation will be more balanced, but cyanosis will be evident. In limited cases, progressive narrowing at the bulboventricular foramen results in significant left ventricular outflow obstruction.

Therapy
Infants with this lesion may be surgically palliated by the single ventricular approach. The first stage usually involves augmenting pulmonary blood flow by a modified Blalock-Taussig shunt[1] with oversewing of the pulmonary artery, and bypassing the potential obstruction at the bulboventricular foramen by a Damus-Kaye-Stansel procedure.[2] If no pulmonary stenosis is present, then pulmonary artery banding[3] may be done. However, pulmonary banding must be used cautiously as this may result in progressive narrowing of the bulboventricular foramen and systemic ventricular outflow obstruction. The second stage is frequently the Glenn Procedure[4], followed by the final surgical palliation, a modified Fontan procedure.[5]

---

[1] See page 246 for modified Blalock-Taussig Shunt.

[2] See page 252 for Damus-Kaye-Stansel Procedure.

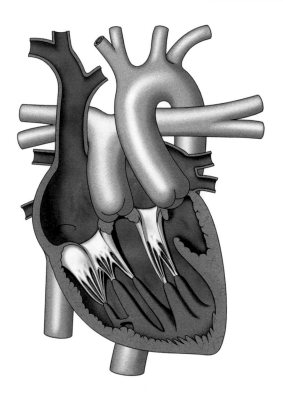

Above: Double-inlet left ventricle

Note following features: Rudimentary right ventricle (bulboventricle); Bulboventricular foramen; transposition of the great arteries; double inlet left ventricle; Atrial septal defect (ASD); ventricular inversion (positions reversed from normal); subpulmonary stenosis due to conal muscle tissue

---

[3] See page 282 for pulmonary artery banding.

[4] See page 262 for the Glenn Procedure.

[5] See pages 258 and 260 for the Fontan Procedure.

Double-Outlet Right Ventricle

Anatomic Description
Double-Outlet Right Ventricle is an uncommon congenital heart defect in which both the aorta and the pulmonary artery arise from the right ventricle. This lesion can also be described as the presence of muscular conal tissue under both pulmonary artery and aorta, with fibrous discontinuity between the aortic and mitral valves. There is a ventricular septal defect (VSD), which can be sub-aortic, sub-pulmonary, doubly-committed, or remote in location. The great vessels may be normally related or transposed in orientation. Rarely, there can be hypoplasia of the mitral valve and left ventricle.

Pathophysiology
The hemodynamic and physiologic effects of this lesion depend on the position of the VSD and the degree of pulmonary valve stenosis. Infants with this lesion may show the spectrum from pulmonary over-circulation to transposition-like physiology. Transposition-like physiology occurs with inadequate circulatory mixing due to streaming of oxygenated blood across the VSD from the left ventricle back to the pulmonary artery (Taussig-Bing Anomaly).

Therapy
Surgery is the mainstay of therapy for this lesion. In patients with normally related great vessels and sub-aortic VSD, primary repair can be accomplished by patching the VSD to the aorta. If the aorta is remote from the VSD, a Rastelli-like procedure[1] can be performed to baffle the left ventricular output to the aorta, and a conduit placed to route systemic venous blood from the right ventricle to the pulmonary arteries. In cases associated with hypoplasia of the left heart, single ventricular surgical palliation is required.

Opposite: Double-outlet right ventricle

   Top - with transposed great arteries
   Bottom - with normally related great arteries

   CT - conal tissue, VSD - ventricular septal defect

---

[1] See page 254 for the Rastelli Procedure.

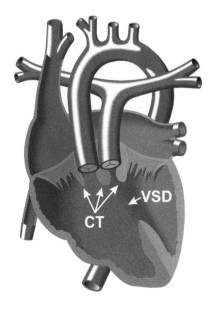

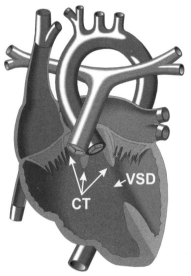

Anatomic Description

This uncommon defect involves an abnormality of the tricuspid valve. It is abnormally formed and is more apically displaced than usual in the heart. This apical displacement of the valve creates atrialization of a portion of the right ventricle. If significant, this abnormal tricuspid valve can be regurgitant, leading to further dilation of the right atrium, which can be severe. In the presence of an atrial communication, there can be right-to-left shunting and resultant cyanosis. In addition, with severe tricuspid insufficiency, there can be functional or developed atresia of the pulmonary valve.

An arrhythmic substrate can be associated with Ebstein's anomaly. This can be due to a manifest accessory electrical pathway, causing Wolff-Parkinson-White syndrome, or due to atrial stretch and fibrosis leading to atrial flutter.

Pathophysiology

The hemodynamic effects of Ebstein's anomaly can vary significantly. In mild cases, patients can be asymptomatic. In more severe cases, the infants present at birth with severe cardiomegaly and cyanosis. The degree of cardiomegaly on the chest x-ray can be impressive, with the massively dilated right atrium causing the heart shadow to fill the entire chest. With severe insufficiency of the tricuspid valve, the right ventricle is unable to generate enough antegrade flow to open the pulmonary valve, leading to functional atresia and ductal dependency.

In some mild cases, the first sign of Ebstein's anomaly may be the finding of pre-excitation on the surface ECG or an arrhythmia.

Therapy

Surgical intervention for Ebstein's presenting in infancy often involves placing a Blalock-Taussig shunt[1] to ensure adequate pulmonary blood flow. For older patients, reparative procedures on the tricuspid valve have been performed, with limited degrees of success.[2] Otherwise, tricuspid valve replacement has been performed.

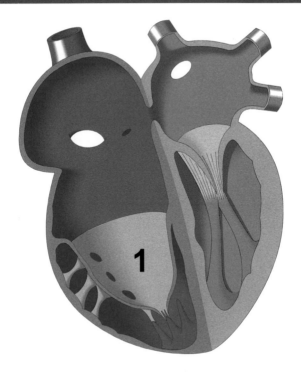

Above: Ebstein's anomaly of the tricupsid valve

1 - Abnormal apical displacement of the tricuspid valve resulting in atrialization of the right ventricle

---

[1] See page 246 for modified Blalock-Taussig Shunt.

[2] See page 256 for Carpentier's Procedure.

Anatomic Description

Abnormal hypertrophy of the ventricular myocardium is often asymmetric, particularly affecting the ventricular septum, and leading to left ventricular outflow tract obstruction. Less severe forms can involve only the apical portion of the left ventricle. Severe obstructive left ventricular hypertrophy is often related to genetic defects of the contractile proteins such as beta-myosin heavy chain.

Pathophysiology

The hypertrophied ventricular septum results in left ventricular outflow tract obstruction, and an increase in afterload on the heart, and worsening compensatory hypertrophy. Significant ventricular hypertrophy leads to diastolic dysfunction of the left ventricle, and an increase in the end-diastolic pressure. The decreased coronary perfusion pressure (from the increased end-diastolic pressure and the decreased diastolic aortic pressure from outflow obstruction) and the increased myocardial oxygen demand, can lead to coronary insufficiency and ischemia. Angina results and limits the patient's exercise tolerance. In severely affected patients, ventricular arrhythmias can develop, and sudden cardiac death can result.

With significant sub-aortic obstruction, the Venturi effect from increased velocity flow out the left ventricle entrains the anterior leaflet of the mitral valve (systolic anterior motion, or "SAM") leading to significant associated mitral regurgitation.

Therapy

Medical therapy has included beta blockers and calcium channel blockers, which decrease myocardial oxygen demand and slow the heart rate, thereby increasing diastolic filling. They, as well as disopyramide, have relieved symptoms in only ~50% of patients.

For those patients with medically refractory symptoms secondary to significant left ventricular outflow tract obstruction, surgical septal myectomy[1] or transcatheter alcohol septal ablation has been performed.

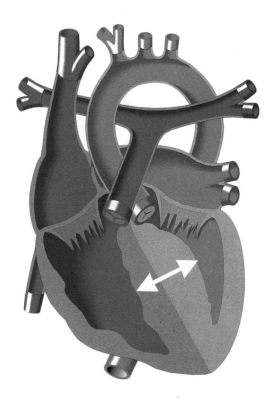

Above – Note asymmetric hypertrophy of ventricular septum and left ventricular free wall.

Because of the risk of sudden death in advanced cases, selected patients are treated with an implantable defibrillator. Ultimately, for patients with severe disease refractory to standard treatment, cardiac transplantation remains a limited option.

---

[1] See page 290 for surgical septal myectomy.

Hypoplastic Left Heart Syndrome

Anatomic Description

Hypoplastic Left Heart Syndrome (HLHS) is characterized by hypoplasia or atresia of the mitral valve, hypoplasia of the left ventricle, aortic stenosis or atresia, hypoplasia of the ascending aorta, and coarctation. There is an atrial septal defect, normally located superiorly on the atrial septum. In rare cases, the atrial defect may be restrictive or the atrial septum may be intact. In those patients, another egress for pulmonary venous blood from the left atrium must exist, such as a decompressing vertical vein.

Pathophysiology

Patency of the ductus arteriosus is obligatory, as this is the main pathway for systemic outflow, including coronary perfusion. The systemic and pulmonary venous blood mixes in the right atrium, creating a mixture of desaturated and saturated blood. However, in the presence of a non-restrictive atrial communication, resistance through the pulmonary circuit will be less than the systemic circuit, and there will be significant pulmonary over-circulation, limiting the degree of cyanosis. In these patients with significant pulmonary over-circulation, congestive heart failure, systemic hypoperfusion, and acidosis may occur.

Infants with a restrictive or intact atrial septum will be both cyanotic and acidotic. Frequently, pulmonary venous abnormalities will coexist, limiting the prognosis of these infants.

Therapy

Initial stabilization with prostaglandins for ductal patency and induction of pulmonary hypertension by careful hypoventilation and occasionally sub-ambient oxygen delivery with nitrogen are required after birth to maintain systemic perfusion. Subsequently, staged surgical palliation or cardiac transplantation have been the treatment options for HLHS. The first stage of surgical palliation is the Norwood Procedure[1] or the Sano Modification[2] of the Norwood Procedure, followed by the Glenn[3] or Hemi-Fontan procedures[4], and culminating in the Fontan procedures.[5]

Recently, some institutions have also used novel transcatheter techniques for the first and third stages of palliation.

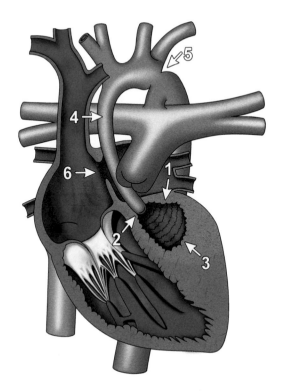

Above: Hypoplastic left heart syndrome

1. Atretic or stenotic mitral valve
2. Atretic or stenotic aortic valve
3. Hypoplastic left ventricle
4. Hypoplastic ascending aorta
5. Coarctation of the aorta
6. Atrial septal defect

---

[1] See page 276 for the Norwood Procedure.
[2] See page 288 for the Sano Modification of the Norwood.
[3] See page 262 for the Glenn Procedure.
[4] See page 264 for the Hemi-Fontan Procedure.
[5] See pages 258 and 260 for the Fontan Procedure.

Interrupted Aortic Arch

Anatomic Description
Interrupted aortic arch can be thought of as the extreme end of the spectrum of coarctation of the aorta, involving a discontinuity between the ascending and descending aorta. There are the obligate additional lesions of a ventricular septal defect and a patent ductus arteriosus. The ventricular septal defect associated with interrupted aortic arch is due to posterior malalignment of the conal septum. Depending on the degree of posterior malalignment, significant left ventricular outflow tract obstruction can occur.

Interruption of the aorta can occur distal to the left subclavian artery (**Type A, opposite**), between the left carotid and left subclavian arteries (**Type B**), or between the innominate and left carotid arteries (**Type C**). Aberrant origin of the right subclavian artery can occur in this lesion, arising as the last branch of the transverse arch. Type B is most commonly associated with thymic agenesis or DiGeorge Syndrome.

Pathophysiology
Prior to ductal closure, infants will have normally saturated blood perfusing the upper body and deoxygenated blood perfusing the lower body, presenting a picture of differential cyanosis. Closure of the ductus arteriosus results in congestive heart failure and inadequate perfusion of the lower body. If not reversed promptly with prostaglandin palliation, profound shock and death results.

Therapy
Prostaglandin E1 is required to maintain ductal patency until surgical intervention. Surgery involves excision of ductal tissue and re-anastomosis of the interrupted portions of the arch.[1] Repair of the ventricular septal defect may be accomplished directly if the left ventricular outflow tract is of adequate size. In cases of significant left ventricular outflow tract obstruction, a complex combination of the Norwood[2] and Rastelli[3] procedures may be performed.

---

[1] See page 266 for surgical repair of IAA.

[2] See page 276 for the Norwood Procedure.

[3] See page 254 for the Rastelli Procedure.

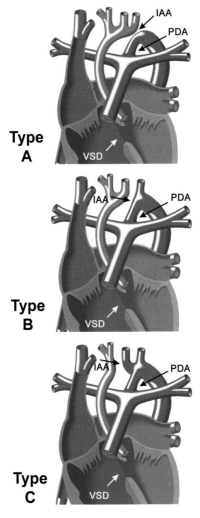

Above - Types of Interrupted aortic arch

    IAA – interrupted aortic arch
    PDA – patent ductus arteriosus
    VSD – ventricular septal defect

Anatomic Description

This acquired heart disease, first described by Dr. Tomisaku Kawasaki in 1967, affects children, with most cases occurring between the ages of 18 and 24 months. Its cause is unknown. A systemic inflammatory state occurs acutely, but the long-term sequelae can lead to arterial aneurysms. Coronary aneurysms are the feared complications. Kawasaki Disease affects boys more commonly than girls (1.5 to 1) and affects Asians (especially Japanese) and children of Asian heritage more frequently than other races.

Pathophysiology

The onset of Kawasaki Disease is marked by a sudden high fever that lasts for at least 5 days. This is accompanied by extreme irritability - more than would be expected from the fever alone. Other systemic findings include edema of the digits, a polymorphous exanthema, a non-purulent conjunctivitis, oral mucosal changes, and cervical lymphadenopathy.

Coronary aneurysms may develop in approximately 20% of untreated cases and less than 5% of treated cases. Coronary aneurysms predispose the affected coronary system to obstruction, thrombosis, and, rarely, vessel rupture.

Therapy

Aspirin and intravenous gamma globulin have been shown to decrease the late incidence of coronary aneurysms, especially if administered during the first 10 days of the illness.

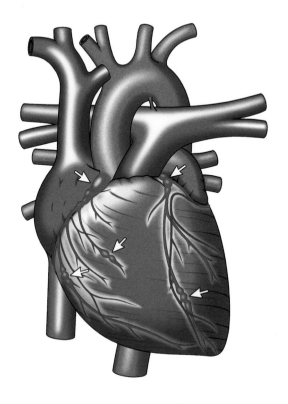

Above: Kawasaki disease, with coronary aneurysms indicated by arrows

Anatomic Description

This inherited genetic abnormality (autosomally dominant) may result in enlargement of the aorta, aortic regurgitation and mitral valve prolapse with insufficiency. The aortic enlargement begins at the sinuses of Valsalva (SV in diagram **opposite**) and extends to the ascending aorta and transverse arch.

Marfan Syndrome was first described by Dr. Antonin Marfan in 1896. It is caused by a broad range of mutations in the fibrillin gene, which occurs in approximately 1 of every 10,000 people. Associated non-cardiac defects include scoliosis, joint laxity, and dislocation of the lens of the eye, and, rarely, skeletal muscle weakness and emphysematous-like lung disease.

Pathophysiology

Marfan is a connective tissue disease with a spectrum from mild aortic dilation to severe ascending aortic aneurysm formation. Aortic dilation is often progressive with risk for aortic dissection and rupture.

Therapy

Aortic dilation is asymptomatic until aortic dissection occurs and therefore requires close follow up to monitor aortic size by echocardiography or cardiac magnetic resonance imaging. Beta-adrenergic blockers or angiotensin II receptor blockers, although not curative, may slow progressive aortic dilation. If the thoracic aorta becomes > 5 cm in diameter, surgical aortic root replacement[1] has been recommended. Mitral valve repair is also quite common. Patients with aortic dilation are frequently exercise restricted because of the concern of aortic dissection.

---

[1] See page 270 for aortic root replacement surgery.

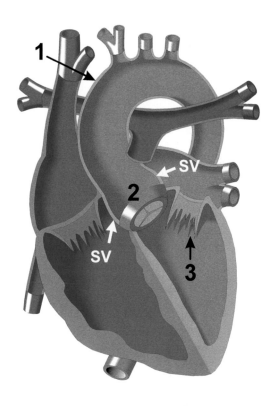

Above: Marfan syndrome

    1. Enlarged ascending aorta
    2. Stretched aortic valve
    3. Mitral valve prolapse
    SV – Sinuses of Valsalva

Anatomic Description

In congenital Mitral Stenosis, the mitral valve leaflets form abnormally. Typically the mitral valve annulus is small with thickened valve leaflets. In some cases, the chordae of the mitral valve will only attach to a single papillary muscle (parachute mitral valve) rather than two, limiting the valve orifice and resulting in stenosis. Non-congenital mitral stenosis is most often a consequence of Rheumatic Fever. In either case, left atrial dilatation occurs.

Pathophysiology

Mitral stenosis, depending on severity, results in elevated left atrial and pulmonary venous pressures.[1] As a consequence, pulmonary hypertension develops with progression to pulmonary edema and right heart failure. With chronic mitral stenosis and left atrial hypertension, atrial dysrhythmias can occur, which increases symptoms and morbidity.

Therapy

Symptoms of pulmonary edema are commonly improved with diuretic therapy. However, patients with significant congenital mitral stenosis should have surgical mitral valve repair[2] or replacement.[3] Rheumatic mitral stenosis can also be palliated by percutaneous mitral balloon valvuloplasty.[4]

---

[1] See page 159, Figure 9B for hemodynamic tracings.

[2] See page 272 for surgical mitral valve repair.

[3] See page 274 for surgical mitral valve replacement.

[4] See page 190 for mitral balloon valvuloplasty.

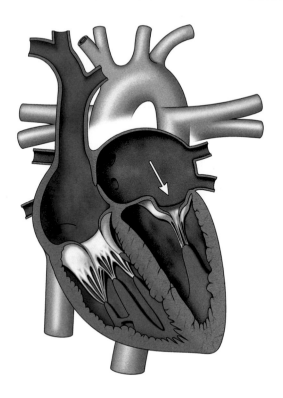

Above: Mitral stenosis (arrow shows abnormally narrow
   mitral valve opening)

Anatomic Description

In Mitral Valve Prolapse, the mitral valve leaflets balloon (prolapse) into the left atrium in systole. Mitral Valve Prolapse may be associated with mitral insufficiency of varying degrees. It is commonly associated with Marfan Syndrome (see page 78) and occurs in otherwise normal individuals.

Pathophysiology

In most cases, a mid-systolic ejection click and, in some, a late diastolic murmur of mitral insufficiency can be heard. Though Mitral Valve Prolapse is usually not serious, patients may describe shortness of breath, palpitations, or chest pain. The etiology of these symptoms is unclear.

Therapy

Mitral Valve Prolapse usually does not require therapy unless significant mitral insufficiency is present.[1,2] Patients with recurrent chest pain will often have symptomatic improvement with beta-blocker therapy.

---

[1] See page 272 for surgical mitral valve repair.

[2] See page 274 for surgical mitral valve replacement.

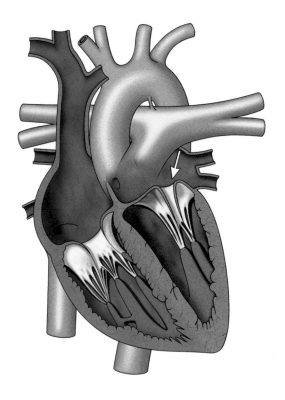

Above: Mitral valve prolapse (prolapsed mitral valve indicated by arrow)

Patent Ductus Arteriosus

Anatomic Description

The Ductus Arteriosus, a branchial arch derivative, connects the main pulmonary artery to the descending aorta. In the fetus, the Ductus Arteriosus shunts blood from the main pulmonary artery to the descending aorta, bypassing the nonaerated lungs. The Ductus Arteriosus normally closes hours after birth with the onset of breathing. Patency of the Ductus Arteriosus in utero is maintained by circulating prostaglandins. After the Ductus Arteriosus closes, it results in the fiber-like structure known as the ligamentum arteriosum. Patent Ductus Arteriosus (PDA) is common in premature infants.

Pathophysiology

As pulmonary vascular resistance is lower in the lungs after birth, a PDA results in a left-to-right shunt from the aorta into the pulmonary artery. If the PDA is large, then heart failure can result from pulmonary overcirculation and pulmonary hypertension. If the PDA is small, the shunt will be insignificant and endocarditis the only risk. A PDA can often be heard as a continuous murmur at the left upper sternal border. In some congenital heart defects (e.g. Pulmonary Atresia, Hypoplastic Left Heart Syndrome, etc.), the PDA is necessary after birth to provide pulmonary or systemic blood flow. Children with these defects (known as "ductal-dependent lesions") require administration of prostaglandin E1 to maintain ductal patency.

Therapy

In the premature infant, if the PDA remains open, pharmacologic treatment with indomethacin or ibuprofen may be used to facilitate closure. If the PDA still does not close, surgical intervention may be necessary. Most isolated PDAs in older infants and children can now be closed in the cardiac catheterization laboratory by coil embolization or other device methods.[1] Surgical closure is by ligation[2] or, alternatively, a metallic clip can be utilized to interrupt the duct.

---

[1] See page 170*ff* for device closures.
[2] See page 278 for surgical ligation.

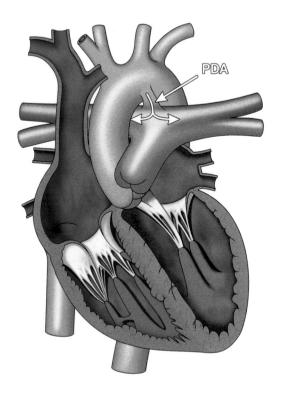

Above: Patent ductus arteriosus (PDA) (direction of blood flow into the pulmonary artery indicated by arrows)

Anatomic Description

In Pulmonary Atresia with Intact Ventricular Septum, the pulmonary valve fails to form properly relatively late in fetal development. As a result, the other two primary components of the right heart, the right ventricle and tricuspid valve, are usually hypoplastic. However there still is a tri-partite (inflow, body, and outflow) right ventricle which may be suitable for a biventricular outcome. Severe hypoplasia of the right ventricle can result in fistulous connections from the right ventricle to the coronary arteries, known as coronary artery sinusoids. The coronary circulation may be dependent on these sinusoidal connections. A patent foramen ovale (PFO) or atrial septal defect (ASD) is present to decompress the obstructed right atrium.

Pathophysiology

In Pulmonary Atresia, pulmonary blood flow is dependent on patency of the Ductus Arteriosus, ensuring a left-to-right shunt. The obligate right-to-left shunt at the atrial septum results in systemic cyanosis. Coronary perfusion of portions of the myocardium may be dependent on the high driving pressure from the obstructed right ventricle via sinusoidal connections. In such cases, anything to decompress the right ventricle (i.e. opening up the atretic pulmonary valve or catheter-induced tricuspid regurgitation) leads to life-threatening ischemia.

Therapy

After diagnosis, Prostaglandin E1 should be administered to maintain ductal patency. In patients with right ventricular dependent coronary sinusoids and a restrictive atrial septum, balloon atrial septostomy[1] may be necessary to produce a large ASD and decompress the right atrium. In the absence of right ventricular dependent coronary sinusoids, primary repair can be accomplished by opening the atretic pulmonary valve. This can be accomplished by transcatheter perforation or surgical valvotomy. In many patients, an additional source of pulmonary blood flow (either a surgically placed aortopulmonary shunt or stenting the patent ductus) is required until right ventricular compliance improves.

---

[1] See pages 162*ff* for balloon atrial septostomy.

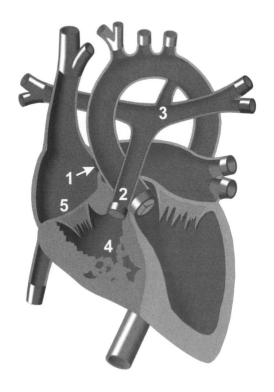

Above: Pulmonary atresia with intact ventricular septum

1. Atrial septal defect
2. Atretic pulmonary valve
3. Patent ductus arteriosus
4. Hypoplastic right ventricle
5. Hypoplastic tricuspid valve

Anatomic Description

Pulmonary atresia with ventricular septal defect is also described as Tetralogy of Fallot with pulmonary atresia, and is thought by many to be an extreme form of the Tetralogy spectrum. In this lesion, no significant right ventricular outflow tract or main pulmonary artery develops. Branch pulmonary arteries may be confluent, fed by a ductus, or may be hypoplastic and discontinuous. In patients with discontinuous pulmonary arteries, frequently no ductus arteriosus is present, but the pulmonary blood flow is provided by aortopulmonary collateral vessels. A large malalignment ventricular septal defect is present, and an atrial septal defect may be present.

Pathophysiology

Complete intracardiac mixing at the atrial and ventricular levels results in systemic desaturation. The natural history of aortopulmonary collateral vessels in this disease is usually one of progressive stenosis and hypoxemia. Frequently, the "true pulmonary arteries" are quite hypoplastic as well.

Therapy

In patients with confluent branch pulmonary arteries fed by a ductus, complete surgical repair in infancy consists of placement of an RV-PA conduit and VSD closure.[1] In patients with multiple hypoplastic aorto-pulmonary vessels, surgical approaches are varied and difficult. Palliative, non-operative care is recommended in some centers. Operative approaches can include pulmonary artery unifocalization with either an aortopulmonary shunt or right ventricular outflow tract reconstruction with a staged incorporation of aorto-pulmonary collaterals into the right ventricular conduit. Eventual closure of the VSD after right ventricular outflow tract reconstruction is dependent on adequate recruitment of pulmonary arterial components.

---

[1] See page 302 for ventricular septal defect closure.

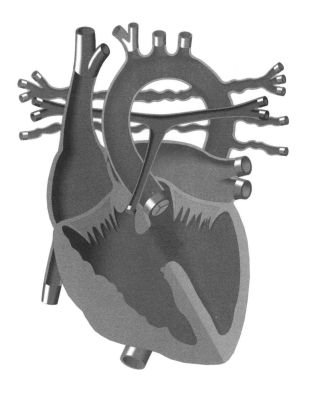

Above: Pulmonary Atresia with VSD showing varied aorto-pulmonary collaterals

Pulmonary Stenosis

Anatomic Description

In this defect, the pulmonary valve opening and/or outflow tract from the right ventricle is restricted. This is one of the more common congenital heart defects and exists as a spectrum from mild to severe.

Types of Pulmonary Stenosis

A. In supravalvar stenosis, the pulmonary artery lumen above the valve opening is narrowed. Obstruction can be in the main or branch pulmonary arteries.

B. In valvar pulmonary stenosis, the leaflets of the pulmonary valve are abnormally thickened and fused at their edges so the valve does not open fully. Often there is poststenotic dilatation of the main pulmonary artery. The valve may be biscuspid or can be dysplastic with redundant tissue.

C. In subvalvar, or infundibular, stenosis, the outflow tract of the right ventricle, below the pulmonary valve, is dynamically obstructed by muscular tissue.

Pathophysiology

Pulmonary Stenosis, unless severe, is well tolerated and children are often asymptomatic. Children with severe stenosis (suprasystemic right ventricular pressure) may develop right sided heart failure. If there is an ASD present, the presence of a stiff, hypertrophied right ventricle leads to decreased compliance and right-to-left shunting with resultant cyanosis.

Moderate pulmonary stenosis (a > 50 mm Hg transvalvar gradient) increases right ventricular pressure and results in the thickening (hypertrophy) of its walls. Even mild pulmonary stenosis results in an easily audible systolic ejection murmur at the left mid to upper sternal border. In general, the higher pitch of the murmur, the greater the stenosis.

Therapy

The course of treatment for this disorder depends on the type and severity of stenosis. Mild stenosis may require no intervention at all. More severe cases may be treated with balloon valvuloplasty[1] (valvular stenosis), angioplasty or stent insertion (branch pulmonary stenosis), or surgical repair.[2]

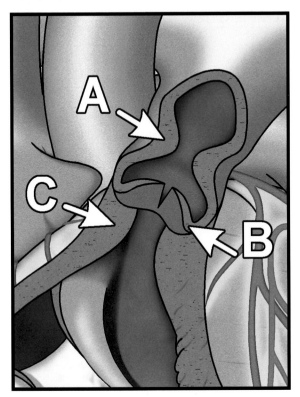

Above: Pulmonary stenosis types

    A. Supravalvar stenosis
    B. Valvar stenosis
    C. Subvalvar, or infundibular stenosis

---

[1] See page 184*ff* for balloon valvuloplasty.

[2] See page 284 for surgical repair of pulmonary stenosis.

Anatomic Description

Tetralogy of Fallot accounts for 10% of the cases of congenital heart disease, affecting both sexes equally. It is the most common cyanotic heart defect beyond infancy and, as the name implies (tetra means four), has four anomalies in its original description:

1. A large anteriorly malaligned ventricular septal defect (VSD) of the conal septum

2. Stenosis of the right ventricular outflow tract (infundibular stenosis) with associated pulmonary valve stenosis

3. The aorta is enlarged and displaced to the right such that it "overrides" the ventricular septal defect.

4. Right ventricular hypertrophy

A right-sided aortic arch (see diagram on page 95) is present in 1/4 to 1/3 of patients. Patients may also have an atrial septal defect.

Pathophysiology

The degree of cyanosis in Tetralogy of Fallot is largely dependent on the degree of obstruction to pulmonary blood flow. Infants with minimal stenosis may have a large left-to-right shunt across the VSD and may have little to no cyanosis ("pink Tetralogy"), while infants with severe right ventricular outflow tract obstruction will be severely cyanotic, with ductal dependent pulmonary blood flow.

Patients with Tetralogy of Fallot may experience intermittent spells of extreme cyanosis, called hypercyanotic spells. These occur because of increased infundibular pulmonary stenosis with stress (crying, dehydration, fever), leading to a worsening cycle of increased right-to-left shunting at the ventricular level and increased cyanosis. Unless reversed, hypercyanotic episodes can be fatal. (continued)

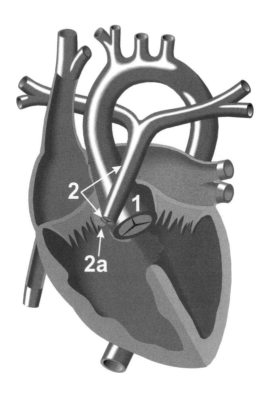

Above: Tetralogy of Fallot

1. Enlarged aorta overriding VSD
2. Stenotic pulmonary valve and artery
2a. Infundibular stenosis

Pathophysiology (continued)

Some patients with Tetralogy may have an associated micro-deletion of chromosome 22, (22q11). Micro deletion of 22q11 is often associated with cono-truncal congenital heart defects (Tetralogy, Truncus Arteriosus and Interrupted Aortic Arch), immune defects and developmental delay.

Therapy

After birth, severely cyanotic infants require a Prostaglandin E1 infusion to maintain ductal patency and pulmonary perfusion. In selected cases, a modified Blalock-Taussig shunt[1] may be performed to provide adequate pulmonary blood flow to the lungs. Depending on the anatomy, complete surgical repair of Tetralogy of Fallot[2] may be successful in the neonatal period but is commonly performed between 4-6 months of age, or with progression of cyanosis. Prior to repair, the right ventricular outflow obstruction in Tetralogy can be progressive, leading to increased cyanosis and risk for hypercyanotic episodes.

---

[1] See page 246 for modified Blalock-Taussig Shunt.
[2] See page 294 for surgical repair of Tetralogy of Fallot.

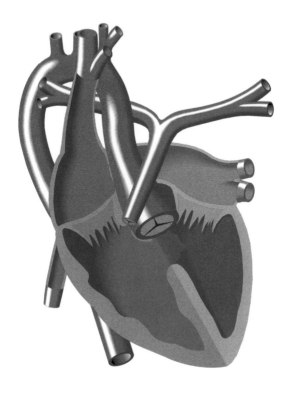

Above: Tetralogy of Fallot with Right Aortic Arch

Anatomic Description

In this defect, which accounts for 5% of the cases of congenital heart disease, the ventricular-arterial relationship is discordant. The aorta is anterior and to the right relative to the pulmonary artery and arises from the right ventricle. Similarly, the pulmonary artery arises from the left ventricle. Associated defects can include ventricular septal defects, pulmonary stenosis, and coarctation of the aorta. Coronary artery anomalies are also common in this defect.

Pathophysiology

In *d*-transposition of the great arteries, the aorta arises from the right ventricle and returns de-oxygenated blood to the systemic circulation while the pulmonary artery arises from the left ventricle and returns oxygenated blood to the pulmonary circulation.

Adequate systemic oxygenation is dependent upon mixing of oxygenated blood from the pulmonary circulation with de-oxygenated blood from the systemic circulation. This occurs at the atrial septum via a patent foramen ovale, and at the great artery level via a patent ductus arteriosus. The atrial communication may be restrictive, leading to significant systemic cyanosis.

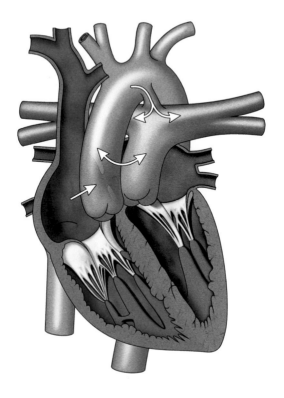

Above: *d*-Transposition of the Great Arteries

Arrows show (left) patent foramen ovale, (center) transposition of arteries, (right) blood flow through the patent ductus arteriosus

Therapy

Soon after birth, the infant is initially palliated by a Prosta-glandin E1 infusion to maintain ductal patency. If the patent foramen ovale is restrictive, inadequate atrial mixing occurs and it must be enlarged by Balloon Septostomy.[1] This defect will require surgery, usually in the first week of life. While the current definitive repair is an Arterial Switch Operation[2], in the past an atrial switch procedure (Mustard or Senning repair) was performed.[3]

Opposite: (views of heart from above)

    Top - *d*-Transposition of the Great Arteries
        LCA - left coronary artery
        RCA - right coronary artery
        AO - Aorta
        PA - pulmonary artery

    Bottom – Normal Heart

---

[1] See page 162*ff* for Balloon Septostomy.

[2] See page 236 for Arterial Switch Operation.

[3] See page 240 for Atrial Switch Operations.

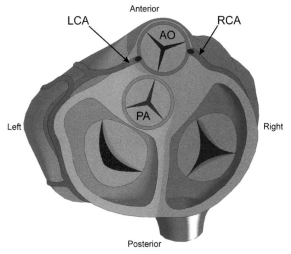

TGA - D

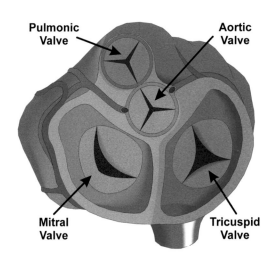

Normal Heart

99

Anatomic Description

l-Transposition of the Great Arteries, or Congenitally-corrected transposition of the great arteries (CCTGA), is an abnormality of atrial-ventricular discordance and ventricular-arterial discordance due to ventricular inversion.

The anatomic right atrium connects to a morphologic right-sided left ventricle via a mitral valve, and has the pulmonary artery as an outlet. The left atrium connects, via the tricuspid valve, to the morphologic left-sided right ventricle with the aorta as the outlet. The aorta lies anterior and to the left of the pulmonary artery.

l-Transposition of the great arteries may be associated with other heart defects including ventricular septal defect and pulmonary stenosis. Uncommonly, *l*-Transposition of the Great Arteries can be associated with right ventricular hypoplasia and single ventricular physiology. It can also be associated with heart block or atrioventricular re-entrant tachycardia.

Pathophysiology

The patient with isolated *l*-Transposition of the Great Arteries may be completely asymptomatic. In some, however, significant tricuspid insufficiency and systemic ventricular dysfunction can occur. In association with a ventricular septal defect and pulmonary stenosis, cyanosis can occur.

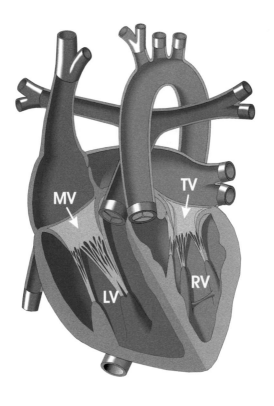

Above: *l*-Transposition of the great arteries - left-sided tricuspid valve (TV) and right-sided mitral valve (MV)

Therapy

For patients with *l*-Transposition of the Great Arteries and significant tricuspid insufficiency or systemic ventricular dysfunction, tricuspid valve replacement has been performed. In selected cases, a "double switch" procedure (a Senning Procedure[1] with an arterial switch procedure) has been attempted to make the morphologic left ventricle into the systemic pumping chamber. However, this complex procedure requires preconditioning of the left ventricle with a pulmonary artery band[2] before it can handle the systemic afterload.

Not infrequently, a pacemaker is required for patients with heart block complicating *l*-Transposition of the Great Arteries.

---

[1] See page 240 for the Senning Procedure.
[2] See page 282 for pulmonary artery band.

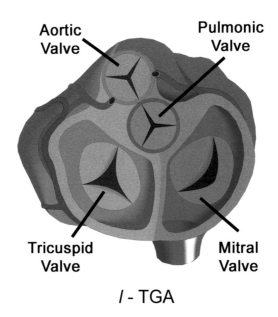

l - TGA

Above: *l*-Transposition of the Great Arteries - View of heart from above. Due to the conus infundibuli the aortic valve is anterior and to the left of the pulmonary valve.

Anatomic Description

The anatomic hallmark of this lesion is absence of the tricuspid valve resulting in complete right ventricular inflow obstruction. An atrial septal defect is always present, and may be restrictive. The great arteries may be normally related or transposed. In patients with tricuspid atresia and normally related great arteries, either a ventricular septal defect is present, or, rarely, pulmonary atresia occurs. In those patients with a ventricular septal defect, varying degrees of obstruction to pulmonary blood flow may occur. In patients with tricuspid atresia and transposed great vessels, coarctation of the aorta or interrupted aortic arch can complicate this defect.

Pathophysiology

There is complete mixing of systemic and pulmonary venous return at the atrial level. Depending on the presence of obstruction to pulmonary blood flow (such as a restrictive VSD with normally related great arteries) infants may be cyanotic or with pulmonary overcirculation in the absence of pulmonary stenosis. In severe cases, infants are dependent upon patency of the ductus arteriosus for pulmonary blood flow. Rarely, the atrial septal defect may become restrictive over time, leading to systemic venous congestion and low cardiac output. Some children with a large VSD and little pulmonary stenosis may have a large left-to-right shunt and require pulmonary banding.

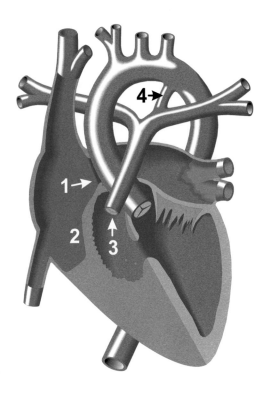

Above: Tricuspid Atresia with ventricular septal defect and
normally-related great arteries

1. Atrial septal defect
2. Atretic tricuspid valve
3. Pulmonary stenosis
4. Patent ductus arteriosus

Therapy

In neonates with either a significantly restrictive ventricular septal defect or pulmonary atresia, prostaglandin E1 infusion is necessary to maintain ductal patency.

Surgical palliation of tricuspid atresia has evolved into a 3 stage surgery. The first stage ensures appropriate pulmonary blood flow, which is often accomplished by a modified Blalock-Taussig shunt.[1] In patients with a moderately restrictive ventricular septal defect, this stage may be cautiously omitted, provided pulmonary arterial pressure is appropriate for later Fontan palliation. The second stage is the bi-directional Glenn[2] or Hemi-Fontan[3] procedures, followed by the third stage of the Fontan procedure.[4]

---

[1] See page 246 for modified Blalock-Taussig Shunt.

[2] See page 262 for the Glenn Procedure.

[3] See page 264 for the Hemi-Fontan Procedure.

[4] See pages 258 and 260 for the Fontan Procedure.

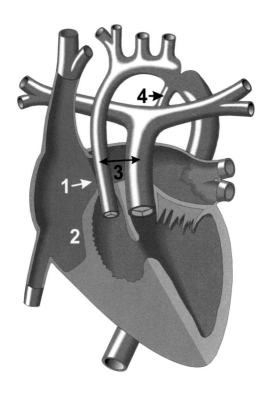

Above: Tricuspid Atresia with VSD and D-Type Transposition of the Great Arteries

1. Atrial septal defect
2. Missing tricuspid valve
3. Transposition of the great arteries
4. Patent ductus arteriosus

107

Truncus Arteriosus

Anatomic Description

In this rare defect, which can occur with other genetic disorders, the aorta and the pulmonary artery leave the heart as a common trunk known as the Truncus Arteriosus. In addition, there is a large Ventricular Septal Defect (VSD), which the Truncus Arteriosus overrides. The pulmonary arteries arise from the Truncus Arteriosus as either a confluent or more commonly, separate origins.

The Truncal valve is often abnormal in form, sometimes with two, four, or five valve leaflets rather than the normal three. The valve can also be both stenotic and insufficient with myxomatous valve leaflets. The aortic arch may be right-sided. Infants with Truncus Arteriosus may also have the associated defects of DiGeorge Syndrome (hypocalcemia, thymic dysfunction and mental retardation) associated with a micro-deletion of chromosome 22, (22q11). Rarely, Truncus Arteriosus is associated with aortic arch or branch pulmonary artery abnormalities.

Pathophysiology

In Truncus Arteriosus, there is complete intracardiac mixing of the systemic and pulmonary venous return, with resultant systemic desaturation. As the pulmonary vascular resistance is less than the systemic vascular resistance, there is usually pulmonary overcirculation and congestive heart failure. Because the pulmonary arteries are exposed to increased flow and frequently systemic pressure, early pulmonary vascular obstructive disease may result.

Therapy

Surgical treatment of this defect involves closure of the ventricular septal defect[1] with detachment of the pulmonary arteries from the common trunk and incorporating them into a right ventricle to pulmonary artery conduit. In patients with significantly stenotic or insufficient truncal valves, surgical repair of the valve has met with limited success, with many requiring replacement with a prosthetic valve.[2]

---

[1] See page 302 for closure of the ventricular septal defect.

[2] See page 296 for replacement with a prosthetic valve.

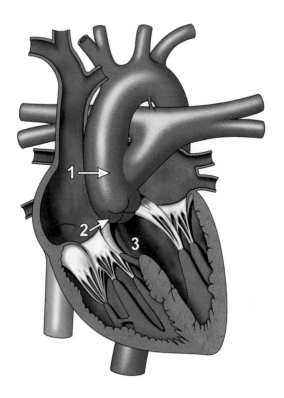

Above: Truncus arteriosus

1. Truncus Arteriosus (Type I)
2. Abnormal truncal valve (4 leaflets)
3. Ventricular septal defect (VSD)

See following pages for other forms of Truncus Arteriosus

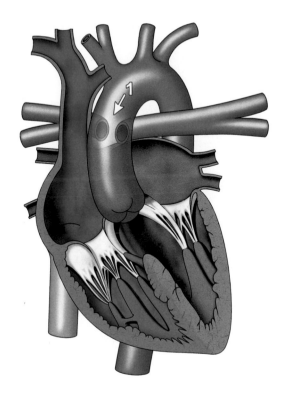

Above: Truncus arteriosus

   1. Truncus Arteriosus (Type II)

   (Note abnormal truncal valve (4 leaflets) and
   Ventricular septal defect (VSD))

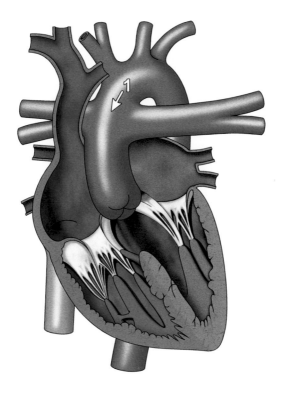

Above: Truncus arteriosus

1. Truncus Arteriosus (Type III)

(Note abnormal truncal valve (4 leaflets) and
Ventricular septal defect (VSD))

Vascular Ring

<u>Anatomic Description</u>

A vascular ring refers to a group of abnormalities of the aorta and its branches. True or complete vascular ring refers to conditions in which abnormal vessels form a complete circle around the trachea and esophagus.

There are two types of complete vascular rings:

1. Double Aortic Arch (see page 114)

2. Right aortic arch with left ligamentum arteriosum (see illustration, **opposite**)

Double aortic arch is the most common vascular ring (40%). Right aortic arch with left ligamentum arteriosum is the second most common vascular ring (30%).

The Double Aortic Arch (page 114) results from the lack of regression of the left side of the embryonic double aortic arch. Persistence of the double aortic arch allows the arch to surround both the trachea and esophagus. A barium swallow would demonstrate high right and lower left lateral indentions into the barium column, representing the compression caused by the right and left arches.

The next most common version of a vascular ring (**opposite**) requires a right aortic arch. The course of the right aortic arch allows the left subclavian artery to wrap around behind the esophagous (retroesophageal left subclavian artery) as it crosses from right to left. There may also be an enlargement of the origin of the left subclavian artery wall, known as Kommerell's diverticulum, in the vicinity of the trachea. This results in trachea constriction. The ring is completed by a left-sided patent ductus or ligamentum.

On a barium swallow, a posterior indention will be seen in the barium column demonstrating the compression by the Kommerell's diverticulum/retroesophageal left subclavian artery.

112

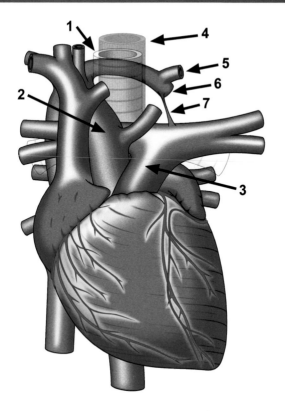

Above: Vascular ring

1. Trachea
2. Aorta
3. Pulmonary artery
4. Esophagus
5. Subclavian artery
6. Kommerell's Diverticulum
7. Ligamentum Arteriosum

Pathophysiology

The symptoms associated with this defect involve the compression of the trachea and esophagus by the surrounding vascular ring. Airway obstruction may occur as the trachea is compressed, resulting in inspiratory stridor. The esophageal compression may result in dysphagia, which may be pronounced with solid food.

Therapy

Treatment of this defect involves removal of the smaller portion of the double aortic arch[1] or the division of the ligamentum arteriosum in children with right aortic arch and a vascular ring. In addition, Kommerell's diverticulum may be removed from the left subclavian artery, which is then closed with sutures.[2] These procedures sever the constricting ring around the trachea and esophagus.

Opposite: Double Aortic Arch

> **Top** - Double Aortic Arch with trachea (light gray) and esophagus (dark gray)

> **Bottom** - Double Aortic Arch with esophagus and trachea removed

---

[1] See page 298 for ligation and division of the smaller portion of the double aortic arch.

[2] See page 300 for removal of Kommerell's diverticulum.

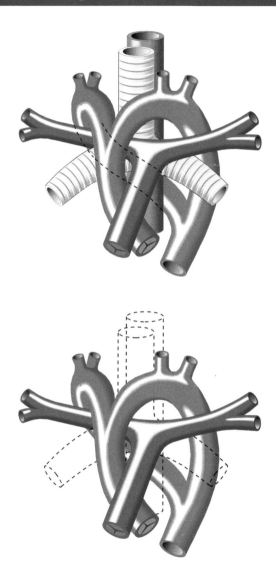

115

Ventricular Septal Defect

Anatomic Description

A Ventricular Septal Defect (VSD) is a myocardial defect in the ventricular septum.

Ventricular septal defects are some of the most common forms of congenital heart disease, accounting for 21% of all cases. They may be single or multiple, and may occur in multiple locations in the ventricular septum (inlet, muscular, perimembranous, or supracristal - see page 119). Small defects usually close spontaneously in the first few years of life. A large defect is characterized by a significant left-to-right shunt (with subsequent dilation of the pulmonary arteries, left atrium, and ventricle), systemic right ventricular pressures, and a diameter similar to the aortic annulus. A small defect is pressure restrictive, with a small shunt (normal chamber sizes) and is only several millimeters in diameter. Muscular and perimembranous defects can decrease in size over time. Malalignment type defects as seen in tetralogy of Fallot never decrease in size.

The supracristal VSD requires special consideration because its spontaneous closure can involve prolapse of the right coronary cusp of the aortic valve into the defect, with cumulative damage to the aortic valve and aortic insufficiency. This can occur less commonly with perimembranous defects as well.

Ventricular septal defects frequently occur with other heart defects.

Pathophysiology

The ventricular septal defect allows the shunting of blood between the ventricles. Most commonly, oxygenated blood shunts from the left ventricle across the defect to the right ventricle. If the left-to-right shunt at the ventricular level is significant, there is excessive pulmonary blood flow resulting in pulmonary edema and tachypnea. Increased pulmonary venous return results in left atrial and ventricular enlargement.

A holosystolic murmur is heard at the left lower sternal border as a result of turbulent blood flow crossing the defect.

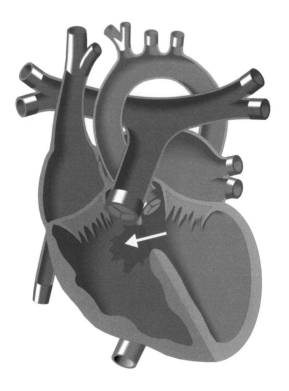

Above: *Ventricular Septal Defect*

White arrow indicates the direction of blood flow through the ventricular septal defect - a left to right shunt.

Pathophysiology (continued)
In smaller defects, the murmur is of higher pitch. The shunt
from smaller defects generally causes little or no hemodynamic effect. Larger shunts may interfere with a child's feeding and growth and may cause rapid breathing, irritability,
excessive sweating, and poor weight gain.

Exposure of the lungs to increased flow and high pressure
from a large VSD over years can result in irreversible pulmonary hypertension and pulmonary vascular obstructive-
disease, with resultant right-to-left shunting (Eisenmenger's
Syndrome).

Therapy
Infants with congestive heart failure because of volume overload to the lungs may be treated with diuretics. As infants
with congestive heart failure have increased metabolic re-
quirements and impaired feeding, high calorie formulas are
often necessary to maximize growth. If impaired growth and
other symptoms persist, surgery is indicated to close the ventricular septal defect.

VSDs can be closed surgically by patch repair.[1] Small defects
may be closed with simple suturing of the edges of the defect.

Surgical repair of muscular defects may be difficult because
the defects are sometimes obscured by the trabeculations of
the right ventricle.

The development of percutaneous device closure of muscular
ventricular septal defects may supplant surgery in selected
cases.[2]

---

[1] See page 302 for patching of ventricular septal defects.

[2] See page 178*ff* for device closure of ventricular septal
defects.

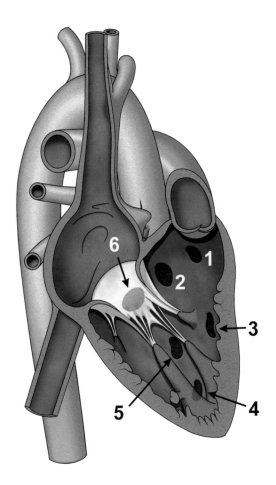

Above: Types of ventricular septal defects

1. Supracristal/outlet
2. Perimembranous
3. Anterior muscular
4. Apical
5. Mid-muscular
6. Inlet

CHAPTER 3. **ECHOCARDIOGRAPHY**

By Howard P. Gutgesell, MD

Two-Dimensional Echocardiography

Two-dimensional echocardiograms illustrate tomographic slices through the heart and great arteries. Although an infinite number of imaging planes are possible, most echocardiograms are obtained from a standardized set of transducer positions. The illustrations which follow show the commonly used transducer positions and the various imaging planes available from that location, the internal anatomy of the heart as seen from each of these planes, and an actual two-dimensional echocardiogram obtained in that imaging plane.

Left Parasternal Long Axis

The transducer is in the 3rd or 4th interspace just to the left of the sternum. The imaging plane transsects the aortic root, the left ventricular outflow tract, and the body of the left ventricle. The image is typically viewed from the patient's left side, head to the right of the screen and feet toward the left. The aortic and mitral valves are well seen. A small portion of the right ventricle is visible anterior to the ventricular septum.

Opposite:

> **Figure 1a** - Imaging plane for the left parasternal long axis projection

> **Figure 1b** - Internal anatomy of the heart as seen from the left parasternal long axis projection

> **Figure 1c** - Representative two-dimensional echocardiogram obtained from the left parasternal long axis projection

> > RV - right ventricle, LV - left ventricle,
> > PA - pulmonary artery, LA - left atrium, Ao - aorta

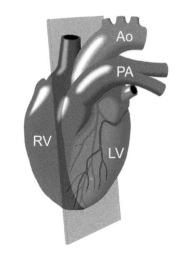

Fig. 1a

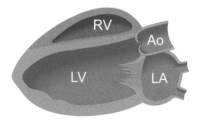

Fig. 1b

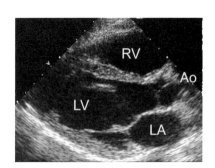

Fig. 1c

123

Left Parasternal Short Axis

With the transducer in the 3rd or 4th interspace but rotated 90 degrees from the long axis view, the left parasternal short axis views slice the heart like a loaf of bread (**Figure 2, below**). The images are viewed as if looking superiorly from the apex of the heart. The most superior plane (**Figure 2a**) shows the aortic root and aortic valve in cross-section. The right ventricular outflow tract and pulmonary valve are seen anterior to the aorta. The main pulmonary artery branches into the left and right pulmonary arteries.

A mid-level plane (**Figure 2b**) passes through the body of the left ventricle. The mitral leaflets have the appearance of a fish mouth when they open in diastole. The left ventricle appears circular.

The most inferior short-axis plane (**Figure 2c**), near the apex of the left ventricle, demonstrates the papillary muscles in the left ventricle.

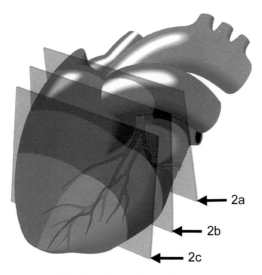

← 2a

← 2b

← 2c

Fig. 2 - Short Axis Planes

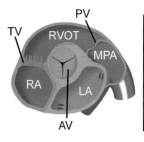 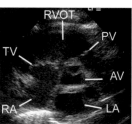

Fig. 2a

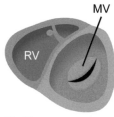 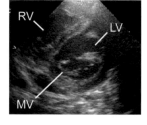

Fig. 2b

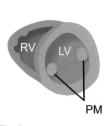 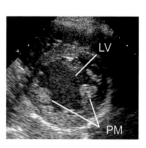

Fig. 2c

AV - aortic valve, LV - left ventricle, MPA - main pulmonary artery, MV - mitral valve, PM - mitral papillary muscle, PV - pulmonary valve, RV - right ventricle, RVOT - right ventricular outflow tract, TV - tricuspid valve

Four-Chamber Views

The four-chamber views (**Figure 3, below**) are obtained from the cardiac apex. The imaging planes slice the heart like a clam shell. The image is oriented with the apex at the bottom (similar to viewing a chest x-ray), as if looking at the bottom half of the clam.

Posterior angulation of the transducer demonstrates the posterior aspect of the mitral and tricuspid annuli and the coronary sinus (**Figure 3a**).

As the transducer is tilted anteriorly, all four chambers and two atrio-ventricular valves are seen (**Figure 3b**).

A shallow, anterior transducer plane transects the aortic valve and left ventricular outflow tract, as well as the mitral and tricuspid valves, both atria and both ventricles (so-called five-chamber view) (**Figure 3c**).

A similar family of four chamber views (not shown) can be obtained from the subxyphoid area in infants and many children. This aligns the atrial and ventricular septa more perpendicular to the ultrasound beam and aids in visualization of defects in these structures.

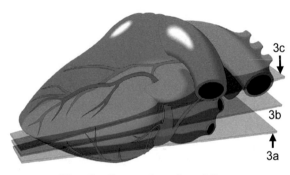

Fig. 3 - Four-chamber Views

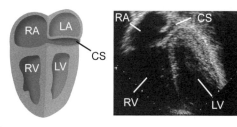

Fig. 3a

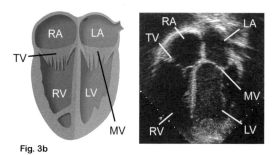

Fig. 3b

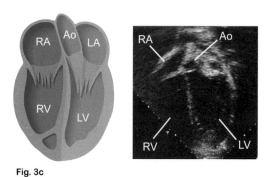

Fig. 3c

Ao - aorta, CS - coronary sinus, LA - left atrium,
LV - left ventricle, MV - mitral valve, RA - right atrium,
RV - right ventricle, TV - tricuspid valve

127

Subcostal Sagittal Views

The subcostal sagittal views (**Figure 4, below**) are perpendicular to the four-chamber views. The transducer is in the subxyphoid region and is rotated about 90 degrees clockwise from the four-chamber views. Like lateral angiograms, they are viewed as if looking from the patient's left side.

The most rightward plane (**Figure 4a**) transects the superior and inferior venae cavae and their connection to the right atrium. The atrial septum is seen in its superior to inferior dimension, and a portion of the left atrium is seen posterior to the septum.

As the transducer is angled toward the patient's left, the beam passes through the body of the right ventricle, its outflow tract, and the pulmonary valve (**Figure 4b**).

Further leftward angulation of the transducer provides a short-axis view of the left ventricle (**Figure 4c**). In the mid portion the mitral valve is seen enface and with still further leftward angulation the papillary muscles are seen.

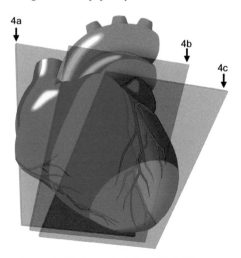

Fig. 4 - Subcostal Sagittal Planes

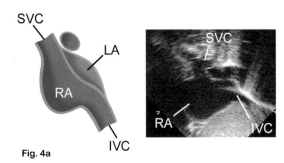

Fig. 4a

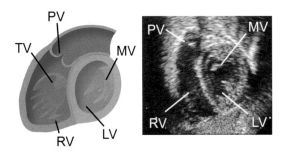

Fig. 4b

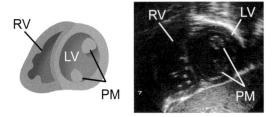

Fig. 4c

IVC - inferior vena cava, LA - left atrium, LV - left ventricle,
MV - mitral valve, PM - mitral papillary muscle,
PV - pulmonic valve, RA - right atrium, RV - right ventricle,
SVC - superior vena cava, TV - tricuspid valve

Abdominal Views

The abdominal sagittal and transverse views, obtained from the subxyphoid region (**Figure. 5, below**), are useful to demonstrate the inferior vena cava, hepatic veins, and abdominal aorta. The sagittal images are viewed as if at the patient's left side, the transverse view from the feet.

A transverse imaging plane through the abdomen shows the liver on the patient's right side and the stomach on the left (**Figure 5a**). A cross-section of the spine is seen posteriorly, with the aorta on the patient's left and the inferior vena cava on the right.

In the sagittal plane (**Figure 5b**), slight rightward angulation of the transducer is used to demonstrate the inferior vena cava passing through the liver and entering the right atrium. Minor angulation will demonstrate the major hepatic veins joining the inferior vena cava just below the right atrium.

Leftward angulation of the transducer provides a longitudinal view of the abdominal aorta (**Figure 5c**). Often the celiac and superior mesenteric arteries can be seen arising from the anterior wall of the aorta.

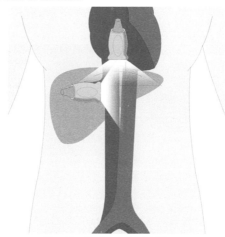

Fig. 5 - Subxyphoid Planes

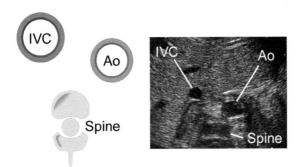

Fig. 5a

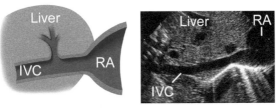

Fig. 5b

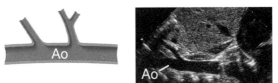

Fig. 5c

Ao - aorta, IVC - inferior vena cava, RA - right atrium

Suprasternal Notch Views

The aortic arch, as well as the ascending and upper portion of the descending aorta, can be imaged from the suprasternal notch (**Figure 6, below**). The images of the long axis of the arch are visualized as if the viewer is in front and slightly to the left of the patient while those of the short axis of the arch are viewed as if in front and slightly to the right of the patient.

The long axis view of the arch demonstrates the ascending aorta, transverse arch, and the upper portion of the descending aorta. The neck vessels can be seen arising from the superior surface of the transverse arch (**Figure 6a**).

The perpendicular plane cuts the transverse arch in cross-section. The innominate vein passes superior to the arch. The right pulmonary artery passes immediately beneath the arch, and beneath it is the left atrium (**Figure 6b**).

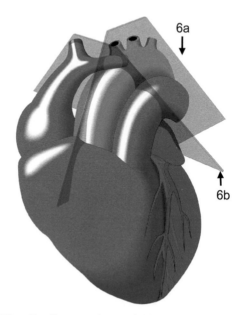

Fig. 6 - Suprasternal Notch Planes

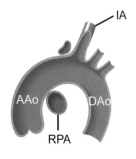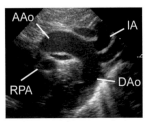

Fig. 6a

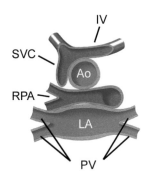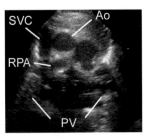

Fig. 6b

AAo - ascending aorta, Ao - aorta, DAo - descending aorta,
IA - innominate artery, IV - innominate vein, LA - left atrium,
PV - pulmonary veins, RPA - right pulmonary artery,
SVC - superior vena cava

133

M-mode Echocardiography

M-mode echocardiograms represent data from a very narrow ultrasound beam plotted against time (an ice-pick view of the heart). These are useful for analyzing patterns of motion of parts of the heart and for measuring the timing of intracardiac events.

The mitral and tricuspid valves abruptly separate at the onset of diastole, begin to float together in mid-diastole, and reopen with atrial contraction, forming a large "M" and smaller "W" pattern (see **Figure 7a, top**). The mid-diastolic closure disappears at faster heart rates. In mitral prolapse the leaflets move posteriorly in mid-systole. In mitral stenosis, the leaflets remain separated throughout diastole.

The aortic valve leaflets are seen between the anterior and posterior walls of the aortic root (see **Figure 7a, bottom**). They separate abruptly with the onset of aortic ejection and close abruptly at the end of ejection. The systolic jet in subaortic stenosis causes the leaflets to vibrate, whereas valvular stenosis is indicated by multiple echoes from the closed leaflets in diastole.

Mitral Valve

Normal HR<140   Normal HR>140

Prolapse

Stenosis

Aortic Valve

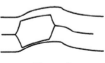

Normal

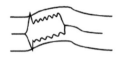

Subaortic Stenosis

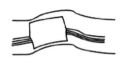

Valvular Stenosis

Fig. 7a

135

M-mode Echocardiography (continued)

Typically, only one of the pulmonary valve leaflets is visualized by M-mode. There is a small posterior dip associated with atrial contraction, followed by an abrupt posterior motion with right ventricular ejection (see **Figure 7b, top**). In pulmonary hypertension, the atrial dip disappears and the leaflet has a "W" pattern in systole.

Recordings made through the body of the left ventricle show the septum and posterior wall approaching each other in systole and separating in diastole (see **Figure 7b, bottom**). As ventricular function deteriorates, the walls become farther apart and their systolic excursion diminishes.

Pulmonary Valve

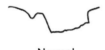

Normal

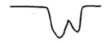

Pulmonary Hypertension

Left Ventricle

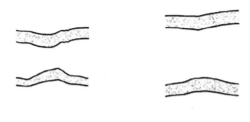

Normal

Dilated, reduced
contractility

Fig. 7b

Doppler Echocardiography

Doppler echocardiography utilizes the change in sound wave frequency produced when the sound wave strikes moving targets (blood cells) to display the direction and velocity of blood flow. Color flow Doppler displays this information as red, blue, or mosaic patterns superimposed upon the two-dimensional echocardiogram. Spectral Doppler displays flow velocity from a single transducer position in a plot against time.

The upper figures on the facing page (**Figures 8a-b**) show color flow Doppler displays. Flow toward the transducer is displayed as red, flow away from the transducer as blue, and high velocity flow is displayed as a mosaic pattern of blue, yellow, and red. In the top image, normal prograde pulmonary blood flow is displayed in blue. The red, yellow, and blue signal represents retrograde flow into the pulmonary artery from a small patent ductus arteriosus. In the lower image, the yellow-blue signal represents mitral insufficiency.

The bottom figure (**Figure 8c**) is a spectral Doppler recording of ascending aortic blood flow in a patient with aortic stenosis. The maximal flow velocity is 3.69 m/s, giving a predicted peak gradient of 54.5 mmHg (obtained using the formula Gradient = 4 x V^2).

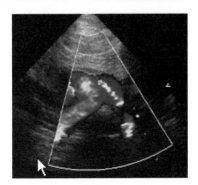

Fig. 8a

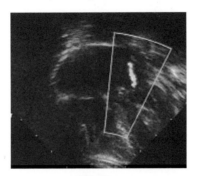

Fig. 8b

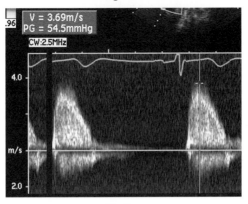

Fig. 8c

Echocardiography - Normal Values

Approximate Upper and Lower Limits of Normal for Echocardiographic Measurements in Pediatric Patients

M-mode	Premature	Premature	Premature	Premature	Newborn	1 yr old	4 yr old	10 yr old	16 yr/Adult
	600 gm	1000 gm	1500 gm	2000 gm	3.5 kg	10 kg	20 kg	35 kg	70 kg
					$0.21\ m^2$	$0.45\ m^2$	$0.75\ m^2$	$1.2\ m^2$	$1.7\ m^2$
LA	3 to 6	4 to 7	5 to 9	9 to 11	7 to 13	12 to 22	16 to 32	20 to 34	24 to 40
LV	7 to 10	9 to 12	10 to 14	12 to 16	15 to 20	24 to 34	30 to 40	34 to 45	42 to 56
Aorta					8 to 12	11 to 18	15 to 24	18 to 27	25 to 35
Septum/ LVPW					3 to 5	4.5 to 6.5	5.5 to 8.5	5 to 9	7.5 to 12
2-D									
Sinuses of Valsalva					10 to 15	12 to 18	13 to 22	20 to 27	24 to 35

LV volume: Approx 45 ml/m² in neonates, increases to 55 ml/m² by 2 yrs, slight increase thereafter		
Annular size: In term infants (3.5 kg, 0.21 m²)		
Mitral annulus 9-18 mm	Mean = 14 mm, each mm smaller = approx 0.5 SD below mean Annulus is 1.3 mm larger for each 1 kg of body weight from 1-4 kg
Tricuspid annulus 9-19 mm	Mean = 14 mm, each mm smaller = approx 0.5 SD below mean Annulus is 1.6 mm larger for each 1 kg of body weight from 1-4 kg
Aortic annulus 5-10 mm	Mean = 8 mm, each mm smaller = approx 1.5 SD below mean Annulus is 1.0 mm larger for each 1 kg of body weight from 1-4 kg
Pulmonary annulus 8-12 mm	Mean = 10 mm, each mm smaller = approx 1.0 SD below mean Annulus is 1.3 mm larger for each 1 kg of body weight from 1-4 kg

Frequently Used Formulas in Echocardiography

M-mode

Shortening Fraction: EDD-ESD/EDD

Vcf: EDD-ESD/EDD x LVET

Vcfc (rate corrected Vcf): EDD-ESD/EDD x LVETc

2-D

LV volume (Bullet): 5 x L x A/6 where L = 4-chamber length from apex to mitral annulus and A = short axis cross-sectional area at level of mitral valve

RV volume: 2 x D x A/3 where D = distance from lateral tricuspid annulus to lateral pulmonary annulus and A = RV area from apical 4=chamber view

Doppler

Pressure gradient (valve): Gradient = $4V^2$

Pressure gradient (aorta or pulmonary arteries):

Gradient = $4 (V_1^2 - V_2^2)$

Myocardial Performance Index (Tei): A – B/ B where A = time from end of mitral inflow to onset of mitral inflow of next beat and B = LVET from outflow signal

2-D and Doppler

Volume of flow: CSA x VTI

Valve area: CSA of outflow tract x V_1/V_2

Abbreviations:

EDD = end-diastolic diameter

ESD = end-systolic diameter

CSA = Cross-sectional area

LVET = left ventricular ejection time

LVETc = LVET/ Square root of R-R interval

VTI = Velocity time integral

V, V_1, V_2 = Velocity, proximal velocity, peak velocity

Quantitative Echocardiography

Findings suggestive of severe Aortic Insufficiency
  Dilation of the LV
  Color jet > 1/3 the area of LVOT
  Pressure half-time < 200
  Pandiastolic flow reversal in thoracic aorta

Findings suggestive of severe Mitral Insufficiency
  Dilation of LV and LA
  Color jet extending to pulmonary veins
  Color jet area > 30% LA area

Grading system for PDA in Prematures
  Trivial: Tiny flow jet (1 or 2 pixels wide)
    LA and LV normal
  Small: Small jet by color Doppler (<25% of PA)
    LA and LV normal
  Moderate: Medium sized color jet (25-50% of PA)
    LA or LV slightly enlarged
  Large: Large color jet (>50% PA)
    LA and LV enlarged

Aortic Stenosis
  Estimation of Cath lab peak-to-peak gradient
    Cath gradient = 6.02 + 1.49 (mean Doppler gradient) - 0.44 (pulse pressure)

  Findings suggestive of severe AS
    Doppler peak gradient > 70mmHg, mean gradient > 30 mmHg
    AVA 0.3 cm^2/m^2

  In neonates
    Decreased LV systolic function
    Development of mitral insufficiency
    Echo-bright papillary muscles

Findings suggestive of Pulmonary Hypertension
    Tricuspid insufficiency jet > 2.7 m/s (RV-RA gradient >30 mmHg)
    PEP/RVET >0.35 (M-mode)
    AT < 40% of ET (Pulsed Doppler)
    Flattening of ventricular septum (2-D short axis)
    PI jet > 2.5 m/s in early diastole (mean PA pressure > 24 mmHg)

Findings suggestive of depressed LV Systolic Function
    Shortening fraction < 28% (M-mode)
    Ejection fraction < 55% (2-D)
    PEP/LVET > 0.4 (M-mode)
    Myocardial performance index (Tei) >0.4
    EPSS > 0.2 mm/mm of LV EDD

Left Ventricular Hypertrophy
    LV mass >120 gm/m^2 (males)
    LV mass > 100 gm/m^2 (females)

References

Lester LA, et al. M-mode echocardiography in normal children and adolescents: some new perspectives. *Pediatric Cardiology* 1987; 8:27-33

Gutgesell HP, et al. Evaluation of left ventricular size and function by echocardiography: results in normal children. *Circulation* 1977; 56:457-462

Gutgesell HP, et al. Growth of the human heart relative to body surface area. *American Journal of Cardiology* 1990; 65:662-668

Henry, WL, et al. Echocardiographic measurements in normal subjects from infancy to old age. *Circulation* 1980; 62:1054-1061

Roge CLL, et al. Cardiac structure growth pattern determined by echocardiography. *Circulation* 1978; 57:285-290

King DH, et al. Mitral and tricuspid valve annular diameter in normal children determined by two-dimensional echocardiography. *American Journal of Cardiology* 1985; 55:787-789

Tacy TA, et al. Range of normal valve annulus size in neonates. *American Journal of Cardiology* 1995; 75:541-543

Roman MJ, et al. Two-dimensional echocardiographic aortic root dimensions in normal children and adults. *American Journal of Cardiology* 1989; 64:507-512

Daubeney, PEF, et al. Relationship of the dimension of cardiac structure to body size: an echocardiographic study in normal infants and children. *Cardiology in the Young* 1999; 9:402-410

CHAPTER 4.
CATHETERIZATION LAB INTERVENTIONS

By D. Scott Lim, M.D.

PERCUTANEOUS VASCULAR ACCESS

Vascular access is the first, and at times, the most difficult and time-consuming part of the cardiac catheterization. Commonly, vascular access to the heart can be accomplished using either the femoral artery or vein, internal jugular vein, subclavian vein, or radial artery. Rarely, access to the cardiovascular system requires a transhepatic venous approach or direct ventricular puncture.

Opposite:

Figure 1 - Vascular access sites

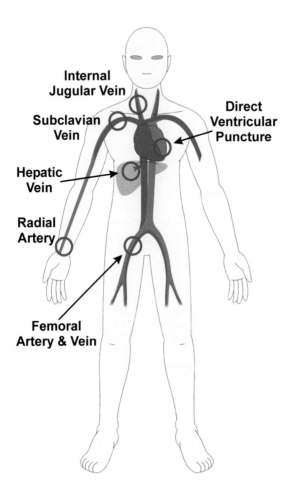

Fig. 1

149

Femoral Vascular Access

Due to the positioning of the patient in the catheterization laboratory as well as relative safety, percutaneous access to the common femoral artery and vein is the site most commonly used in congenital heart disease. Important landmarks to note are the inguinal ligament running between the anterior superior iliac crest and the symphysis pubis. Puncture of the vessel should always be performed well below the inguinal ligament. The neuro-vascular bundle runs underneath this. Access is commonly attempted first in the femoral vein, which is most medial. Initial access to the femoral artery can sometimes distort the anatomy, making subsequent access to the femoral vein more difficult in the smaller patient.

Opposite: Figure 2

Top - Femoral vascular access

Bottom - Angiographic image of femoral artery (FA).

Note that a sheath is in the femoral vein (FV) and demonstrates its usual anatomic location medial to the FA and the femoral head.

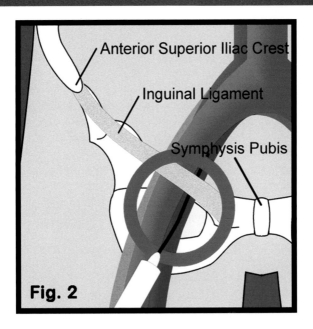

Fig. 2

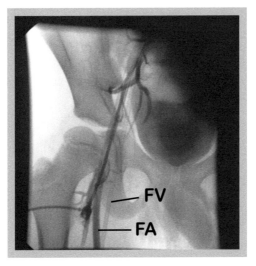

151

Catheterization Laboratory Interventions

Jugular and Subclavian Vein Access

Vascular access using the internal jugular vein (see **Figure 3**) is commonly utilized in patients for endomyocardial biopsy or for those with a superior vena cava-to-pulmonary artery anastomosis. Landmarks include the sternocleidomastoid muscle, manubrial notch, and the carotid pulse. Frequently, the use of ultrasound guidance can assist in obtaining access to the internal jugular vein. Of note, trans-septal access to the left atrium for the use of placing an atrial septal device or antegrade access to the left ventricle, is quite difficult from this approach.

Additionally, access to the superior vena cava can be obtained by the subclavian vein (see **Figure 4**). Predominant landmarks include the bend in the clavicle and the manubrial notch. Access to this vessel is frequently aided by the placement of a support between the patient's shoulder blades. By keeping the entry needle in a relatively flat plane and avoiding cranial or caudal angulation, both inadvertent arterial puncture and pneumothorax can be avoided. Of note, when performing subclavian vein access without use of fluoroscopy, access to the left sided subclavian vein allows for easier tracking of the wire.

Opposite:

> **Figure 3** - Vascular access using the internal jugular vein

> **Figure 4** - Subclavian vein access

152

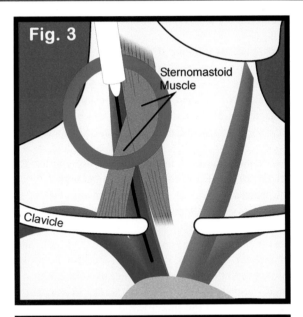

Fig. 3

Sternomastoid Muscle

Clavicle

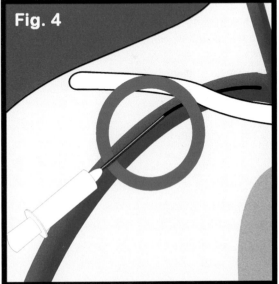

Fig. 4

153

Radial Artery and Transhepatic Access

Arterial access utilizing the radial artery can be done for either pressure monitoring or, in larger patients, arterial access for catheters (see **Figure 5**). Of note, determination of adequate vascular perfusion of that hand by occlusion of the radial artery should be performed before performing radial artery access (Allen's test).

Transhepatic access to the hepatic vessels, and in turn the inferior vena cava, can be performed with relative safety and efficacy (see **Figure. 6**). This procedure involves percutaneous puncture of the liver in the mid-axillary line using fluoroscopy. Once a hepatic vein is identified, a long wire is passed through the needle into the inferior vena cava, over which the sheath can be advanced. At the conclusion of the catheterization, coil embolization of the transhepatic access tract is commonly performed to achieve hemostasis. Of note, transhepatic access is relatively contraindicated in patients with abdominal heterotaxy.

Opposite:

    Figure 5 - Radial artery access

    Figure 6 - Transhepatic access

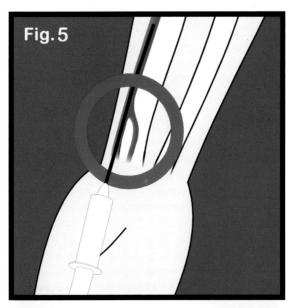

Fig. 5

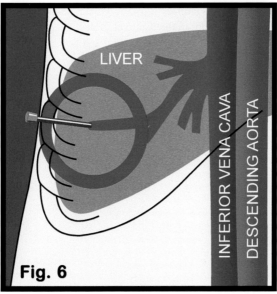

LIVER

INFERIOR VENA CAVA

DESCENDING AORTA

Fig. 6

155

CARDIAC HEMODYNAMICS

Interpreting pressure waveforms in various cardiac chambers is essential to understanding a diagnostic cardiac catheterization. **Figures 8A-F** demonstrate the normal pressure wave forms expected in the respective chambers.

Catheterization measurements are like a jigsaw puzzle in that each recorded pressure tracing from the chamber of interest must make sense with consecutive chamber pressure measurements to create a complete hemodynamic picture. For example, in the absence of atrioventricular valvar stenosis, the A-wave in the atrium must correlate with the end-diastolic pressure in the corresponding ventricle. In the presence of a non-restrictive atrial septal defect, the mean pressure in both right and left atria must be equal. Additionally, in the presence of a competent pulmonary valve, diastolic pressure in the pulmonary arteries must be greater than the end-diastolic pressure in the right ventricle.

Opposite: Normal pressure waveforms

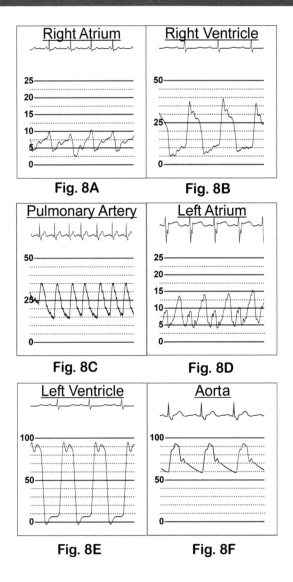

Fig. 8A

Fig. 8B

Fig. 8C

Fig. 8D

Fig. 8E

Fig. 8F

157

Abnormal Pressure Waveforms

Figure 9A shows two pressure tracings, from the aorta and left ventricle, in a patient with aortic valvar stenosis. The peak-to-peak pressure gradient is the difference between the maximum pressure in the left ventricle and the maximum in the ascending aorta. Note that in the patient with aortic stenosis, not only is there a time delay to peak aortic pressure, but the aortic upstroke slope is less steep.

Figure 9B is from a patient with mitral stenosis. In the absence of mitral inflow obstruction, there should be no significant pressure gradient between the left atrium and the left ventricle during diastole. This figure demonstrates a gradient between the "a" wave in the left atrium (atrial systole) and the end-diastolic pressure of the left ventricle.

In mitral insufficiency, it is the "v" wave of the left atrium which is increased by the regurgitant jet, as shown in **Figure 9C**.

Patients with constrictive pericardial disease have impaired diastolic relaxation of the ventricle, with elevated diastolic pressure, as shown in **Figure 9D**. This commonly takes the shape of a "dip and plateau" or "square-root" sign.

Figure 9E is from a patient with significant Aortic Insufficiency and demonstrates a low aortic diastolic pressure. This is due to diastolic run-off back through the aortic valve.

Opposite: Abnormal pressure waveforms

> **Figure 9A** - Aortic stenosis
> **Figure 9B** - Mitral stenosis (ED - end diastole)
> **Figure 9C** - Mitral insufficiency
> **Figure 9D** - Constrictive pericardial disease
> **Figure 9E** - Aortic insufficiency

158

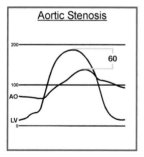

Fig. 9A

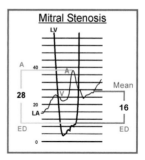

Fig. 9B

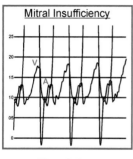

Fig. 9C

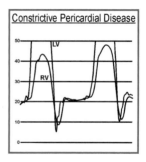

Fig. 9D

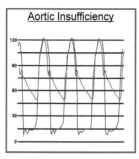

Fig. 9E

ANGIOGRAPHY

Angiography involves placing a catheter in the chamber of interest, and rapidly injecting a quantity of a radio-opaque contrast agent while recording fluoroscopic imagery. Angiography may be performed by hand injection of contrast through an end-hole catheter in the coronary artery, or by power injection into a chamber or vessel of interest, such as the aorta or left ventricle, as shown in figures **10A** (below) and **10B** (opposite).

While the utility of angiography for diagnosis of congenital heart disease has largely been supplanted by noninvasive imaging, biplane cineangiography is a required adjunct to interventional procedures. It is essential to define the pathologic structure of interest by the appropriate angulated views prior to intervention.

Below: Figure 10A - Aortic angiography is performed with caudal angulation to profile the stenotic aortic valve prior to transcatheter aortic valve implantation.

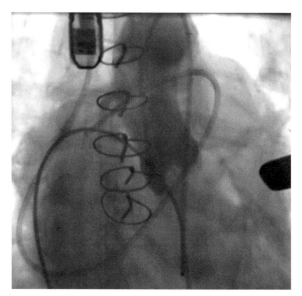

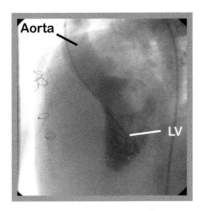

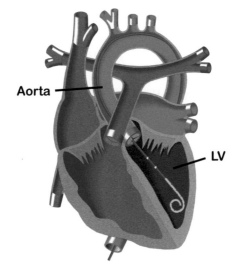

Above: Figure 10B

(Top) Long axis oblique angiographic view of the
left ventricle (LV)

(Bottom) Schematic drawing of pigtail catheter in
the LV (left ventricle), anterior view

161

CONGENITAL CARDIAC INTERVENTIONS

Atrial Septostomy

Creation of an atrial septal defect can be a life-saving procedure, particularly in infants with severe hypoxemia due to *d*-Transposition of the Great Arteries and an intact ventricular septum. The dynamic balloon atrial septostomy is performed by advancing a noncompliant balloon tipped catheter (see **Figure 11**, below, Rashkind-Miller Balloon Atrioseptostomy catheter) from the venous side to the left atrium and rapid pulling or "jerking" the inflated balloon forcibly back across the atrial septum, creating a tear. This then improves inter-atrial mixing of saturated and desaturated blood which is needed in newborns with *d*-transposition of the great arteries and a restrictive atrial septum.

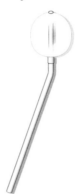

Fig. 11. Rashkind-Miller Catheter

Opposite: Figures 11A-C - Dynamic septostomy

11A - Deflated septostomy catheter advanced across PFO into LA

11B - Inflated septostomy catheter in LA

11C - Catheter with inflated balloon larger than the PFO being forcibly pulled back through the PFO, creating an atrial communication.

RA - right atrium, LA - left atrium,
PFO - patent foramen ovale

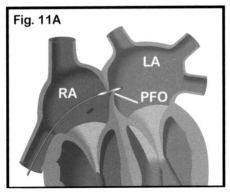

Fig. 11A

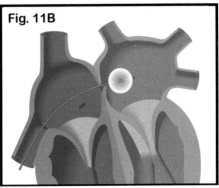

Fig. 11B

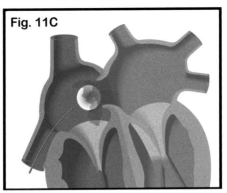

Fig. 11C

Static Balloon

In the older patient with a thicker restrictive atrial septum, either static balloon atrial septostomy (using angioplasty balloons to dilate a defect in the atrial septum), or blade atrial septostomy (see **Figure 14**, page 167) is commonly used.

Opposite: Figures 12A-C - Static septostomy

> **Figure 12A** - Deflated angioplasty balloon catheter advanced across PFO straddling the atrial septum
>
> **Figure 12B** - Inflated balloon catheter across the atrial septum
>
> **Figure 12C** - Catheter with deflated balloon showing the enlarged atrial communication
>
> RA - right atrium, LA - left atrium,
> PFO - patent foramen ovale

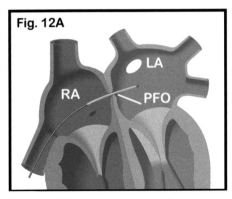

Fig. 12A

RA LA PFO

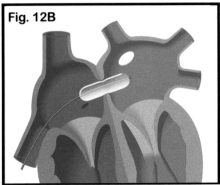

Fig. 12B

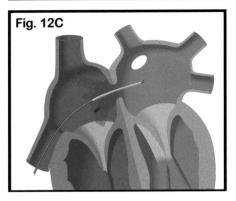

Fig. 12C

Transseptal Puncture and Blade

In non-neonates, both the static balloon and blade atrial septostomies are performed following atrial septal puncture using a Brockenbrough needle in a long sheath (**Figure 13**) or via a radiofrequency perforation wire. The Park blade catheter (**Figure 14**) is then advanced across the atrial septum, and, with the blade deployed, slowly pulled back across the septum creating a cut. Frequently several passes across the atrial septum are performed with the blade angulated differently each time. A blade atrial septostomy is followed by either a static or dynamic balloon septostomy to enlarge the defect. Recently, cutting balloons have also been used to make initial atrial septal cuts prior to balloon septostomy.

Opposite:

> **Figure 13:** Transseptal perforation, using Brockenbrough needle
>
> RA - right atrium
> LA - left atrium
>
> **Figure 14:** Blade septostomy, using Park Blade

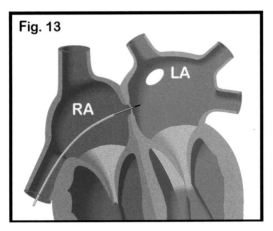

Fig. 13

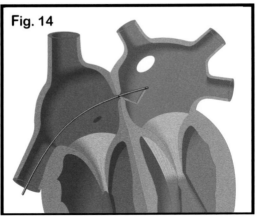

Fig. 14

OCCLUSION OF INTRACARDIAC AND VASCULAR SHUNTS

Occlusion of the patent ductus arteriosus (PDA) is one of the more common procedures performed in the pediatric cardiac catheterization laboratory, (see **Figure 15A**, below).

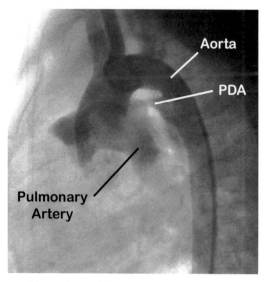

Fig. 15A - PDA Angiogram, Lateral View

The most widely used method is **coil embolization**, which involves placing a stainless steel or platinum spring coil (see **Figure 15B-D**) into the patent ductus arteriosus, inducing thrombosis. Coils can be delivered via a catheter from the arterial or venous side.

Opposite:

> **Figure 15B** - Catheter crossing the PDA from the aortic side and starting to deliver a coil

> **Figure 15C, D** - Coil is fully delivered, occluding the ductus

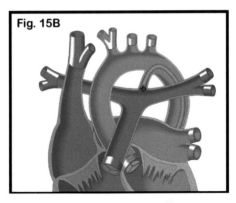

Fig. 15B

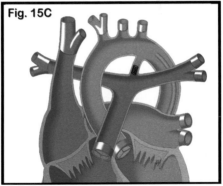

Fig. 15C

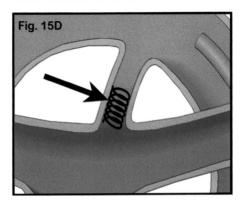

Fig. 15D

Amplatzer Ductal Occluders

The Amplatzer ductal occluder device is a recent addition that allows occlusion of a larger patent ductus arteriosus. This device has a large waist and aortic retention disc and is re-positionable, retrievable and is useful for occluding larger PDA's in patients outside of the neonatal age range. Similarly, a coil-formed device, the Nit-Occlud® by pfm Medical (see **Figure 16A**, below), has found utility in occluding the larger ductus arteriosus.

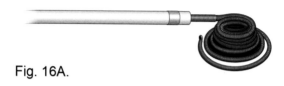

Fig. 16A.

Above:

    Figure 16A - Nit-Occlud® pfm Device

Opposite:

    Figure 16B. Amplatzer ductal occluder

    Figure 16C. Angiogram of PDA occlusion device being delivered, lateral view

170

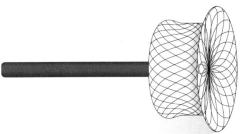

Fig. 16B.

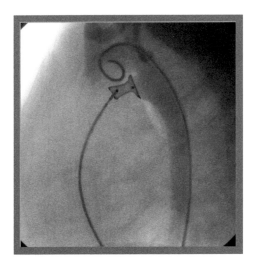

Fig. 16C.

171

Atrial Septal Defect Occlusion

Transcatheter device occlusion has become the therapy of choice for secundum atrial septal defects. Current methods for ASD device occlusion require careful echocardiographic evaluation at the time of defect closure (transesophageal echocardiogram or intracardiac echocardiogram) to determine the rims of the defect as well as stretch balloon sizing of the defect to determine the proper size and type of the device.

Opposite:

> **Figure 17A** - 2D echocardiogram of a secundum atrial septal defect from the subcostal view. The posterior rim and rim near the atrioventricular valves are clearly seen with left-to-right atrial shunting as shown by color Doppler.

> **Figure 17B** - Fluoroscopic image of sizing balloon across an ASD. The indentions in the balloon demonstrate the stretched size of the ASD. The transesophageal echocardiogram probe (TEE) is also seen.

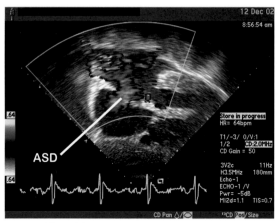

Fig. 17A. ASD Echocardiogram
(Subcostal View)

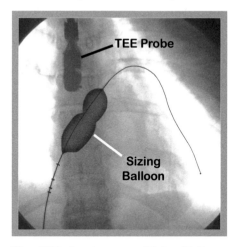

Fig. 17B. Angiogram - Sizing Balloon

173

Currently available devices for transcatheter occlusion of atrial septal defects include the Amplatzer septal occluder, (see **Figure 18A** (below)), STARFlex devices (see **Figure 19B,** page 176), and the Helex device by Gore (see **Figure 18B** (below)).

These devices are delivered from a transvenous approach to the left atrium. The left atrial portion of the device is delivered, and pulled back against the atrial septum. Then, the right atrial portion of the device is delivered. Confirmation of correct device placement is done by fluoroscopy and echocardiography prior to device release.

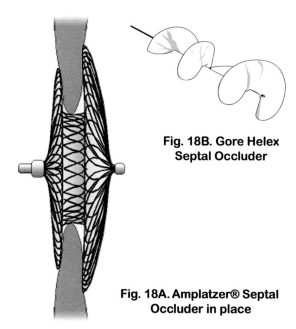

Fig. 18B. Gore Helex Septal Occluder

Fig. 18A. Amplatzer® Septal Occluder in place

Opposite: Figure 18C-E - Occlusion of atrial septal defect with Amplatzer device

RA - right atrium, LA - left atrium, ASD - atrial septal defect

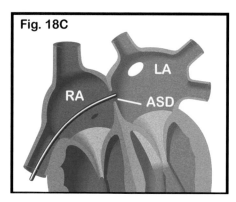

Fig. 18C

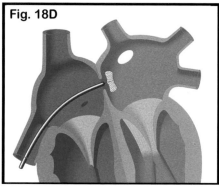

Fig. 18D

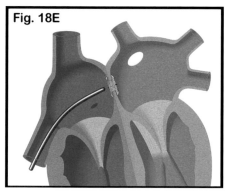

Fig. 18E

Patent Foramen Ovale Occlusion

Transcatheter occlusion of a patent foramen ovale (PFO) has been performed in selected patients to prevent recurrent paradoxical embolism or right-to-left shunting of deoxygenated blood. While no device is generally approved by the US FDA for this primary indication, a number of devices are in various stages of trials, including the Amplatzer PFO occluder, the STARFlex, the Helex device, the Solysafe, and the Premiere devices.

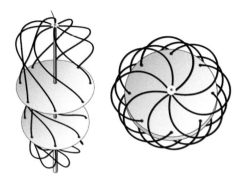

Fig. 19A. Solysafe Septal Occluder

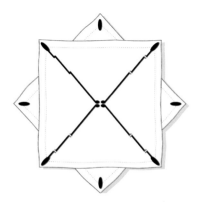

Fig. 19B. STARFlex Septal Occluder

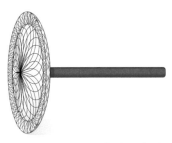

Fig. 19C. Amplatzer PFO Occluder

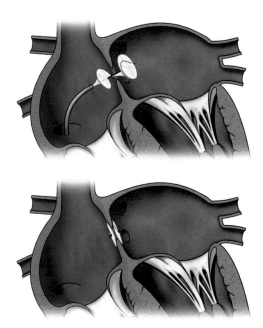

Fig. 19D. Gore Helex Device

Above (bottom): Figure 19D - Transcatheter closure of a patent foramen ovale using a Gore Helex Device

Ventricular Septal Defect Occlusion

Transcatheter therapy for a muscular ventricular septal defect is currently being performed on selected patients. On a very limited basis, this has also been performed on patients with post myocardial infarction ventricular septal defects, but with limited results. Two available devices for this are the STARFlex (see Figure 19B, page 176) and Amplatzer muscular ventricular septal occluder (see **Figure 20C**, opposite).

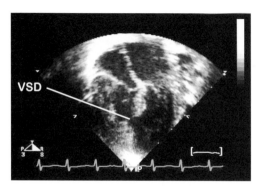

Fig. 20A. Echocardiogram of Muscular VSD

Opposite:

> **Figure 20B-C:** Amplatzer muscular ventricular
> septal occluders

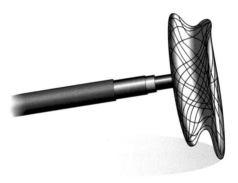

Fig. 20B. Perimembranous VSD Device

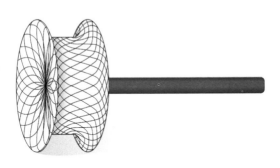

Fig. 20C. Amplatzer VSD Occluder

179

For delivery of VSD devices, a catheter is passed usually from the left ventricle through the defect to the right ventricle and an arterial-venous loop is then formed. This allows deployment of the delivery sheath through the defect from the venous side, through which the device is then delivered (see **Figures 21A-C**). For this procedure, careful transesophageal guidance as well as anesthetic management is mandatory. There has also been successful device closure using a hybrid approach with perventricular access to the heart by a small thoracotomy (see page 216).

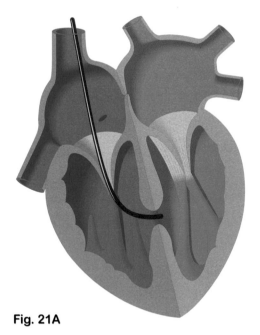

Fig. 21A

Above and Opposite:
Transcatheter delivery of an Amplatzer device from the left ventricle through the ventricular septal defect to the right ventricle

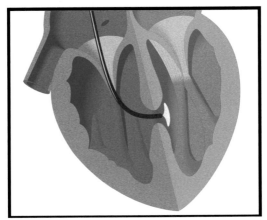

Fig. 21B

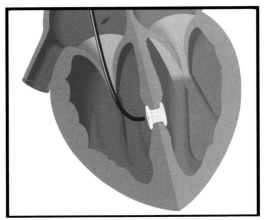

Fig. 21C

181

Fontan Fenestration Occlusion

Transcatheter occlusion of Fontan fenestrations has been utilized with the smaller variants of the septal occluders. Careful angiographic and echocardiographic determination of the fenestration location is required. Frequently the smaller 4 or 5mm Amplatzer septal occluder or the 17mm Cardioseal device is used. From a venous approach, the fenestration is crossed first with an end-hole catheter and then with the delivery sheath. The left atrial portion of the device is deployed, the device and delivery sheath pulled back against the Fontan baffle, and then the right atrial portion of the device is deployed (see **Figures 22 A-B**).

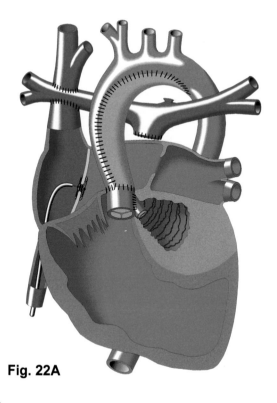

Fig. 22A

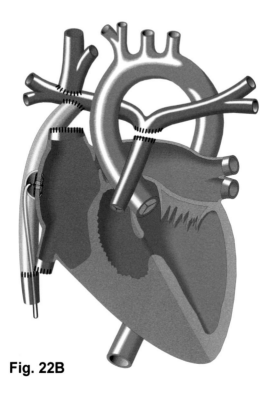

Fig. 22B

Fig. 22B (above): Transcatheter occlusion of an extra-cardiac Fontan fenestration with an Amplatzer septal occluder (tricuspid atresia)

Fig. 22A (opposite): Transcatheter occlusion of a lateral tunnel Fontan fenestration with an Amplatzer septal occluder (hypoplastic left heart syndrome)

183

VALVULOPLASTY

Pulmonary Valvuloplasty

Transcatheter pulmonary balloon valvuloplasty was the first valvuloplasty to be performed with results equal to surgical valvotomy. Paramount to this procedure is the careful determination of pulmonary valve anatomy (stenotic vs. stenotic and dysplastic) by transthoracic echocardiography and pulmonary annulus size, which is done by a lateral right ventricular angiogram.

Opposite:

> **Figure 23A** - Lateral angiogram of stenotic pulmonary valve
>
> **Figure 23B** - Lateral fluoroscopic image of a valvuloplasty balloon inflated across the pulmonary valve

Below: Figure 23C - Pulmonary Stenosis

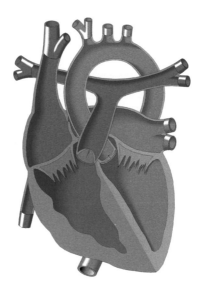

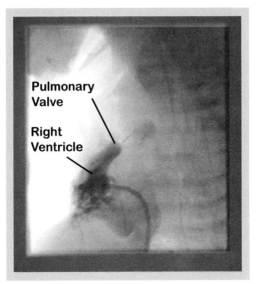

Fig. 23A

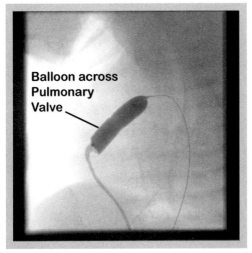

Fig. 23B

185

Size of the balloon used to perform pulmonary valvuloplasty is frequently between 120-140% of the measured pulmonary annulus. This balloon catheter is then passed across the stenotic valve from the venous side and inflated, tearing the stenotic valve leaflets (see **Figure 23B**, page 185 for a lateral fluoroscopic image of pulmonary valvuloplasty).

Opposite:

Figure 24A - Valvuloplasty balloon passed prograde across the stenotic pulmonary valve over a guidewire

Figure 24B - Inflation of the valvuloplasty balloon tearing apart the stenotic pulmonary valve leaflets, relieving the stenosis

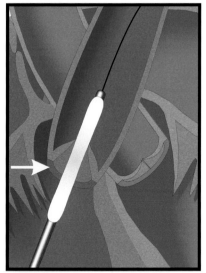

Fig. 24A

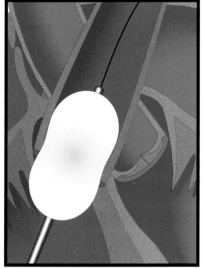

Fig. 24B

187

Aortic Valvuloplasty

Aortic valvuloplasty has been performed, but with greater technical difficulties than pulmonary valvuloplasty. This is due to a need for either an arterial approach or transseptal approach to the left ventricle, resistant valve anatomy, and the need to minimize aortic insufficiency. Again, careful measurement of the aortic annulus is a requirement and frequently the balloon size chosen for valvuloplasty is between 80-100% of the aortic valve annulus to minimize the risk of post-valvuloplasty insufficiency. The valvuloplasty balloon can be passed, either by a retrograde (transaortic) or antegrade (transvenous and transseptal) approach.

Below: Figure 25A - Aortic balloon valvuloplasty is demonstrated and performed by the antegrade (transvenous & transseptal) approach utilizing an Inoue balloon.

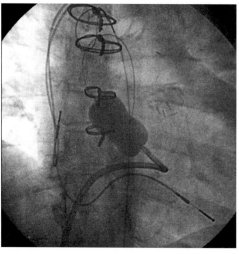

Opposite:

> **Figure 25B** - Valvuloplasty balloon passed retrograde across the stenotic aortic valve over a guidewire

> **Figure 25C** - Inflation of the aortic valvuloplasty balloon tearing apart the stenotic aortic valve leaflets relieving the stenosis

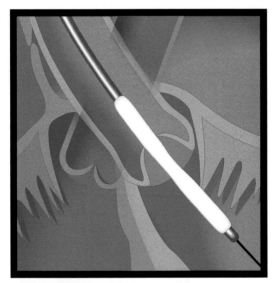

Fig. 25B

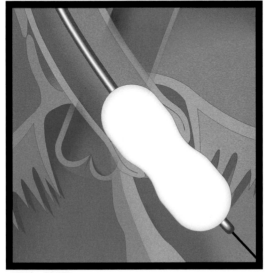

Fig. 25C

189

Mitral Valvuloplasty

In geographical locations where rheumatic valve disease is more prevalent, the use of transcatheter mitral valvuloplasty has remained frequent. This usually involves passing either a single Inoue valvuloplasty balloon across a transseptal atrial puncture into the left atrium and across the mitral valve, or two valvuloplasty balloons side-by-side for inflation and relief of the mitral stenosis. Balloon sizing is based on the height of the patient rather than mitral annulus size.

Opposite:

> **Figure 26A** - Single Inoue valvuloplasty balloon inflated across the stenotic mitral valve.

> **Figure 26B** - Double balloon technique for mitral valvuloplasty across a stenotic mitral valve.

Below: Figure 26C - Cineradiogram demonstrates mitral balloon commissurotomy by the transseptal approach using a single Inoue balloon.

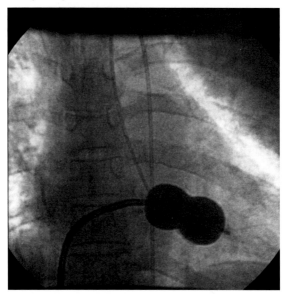

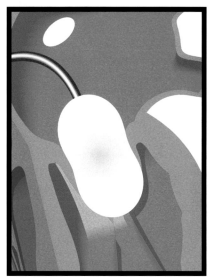

Fig. 26A

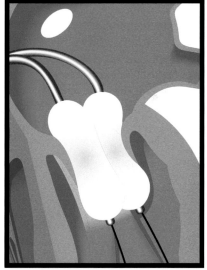

Fig. 26B

ANGIOPLASTY

Pulmonary arterial angioplasty of stenotic branch pulmonary arteries is commonly performed and involves careful pre-procedure angiographic measurement of the stenotic branch pulmonary artery diameters. Following this, a noncompliant angioplasty balloon catheter is passed across the stenotic area and inflated. These catheters frequently involve the use of high inflation pressures, achieved with a pressure manometer. An alternative for small non-compliant arteries is predilation with cutting balloons followed by standard balloon angioplasty.

Opposite:

> **Figure 27A** – Angiogram showing stenotic branch pulmonary arteries
>
> MPA - main pulmonary artery,
> BPA - branch pulmonary arteries
>
> **Figure 27B** – Angioplasty balloon (indicated by arrow) inflated across stenosis seen as an indentation in the inflated balloon

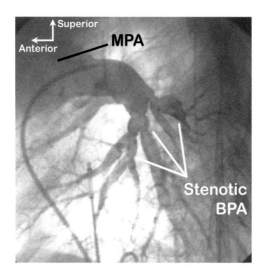

Fig. 27A

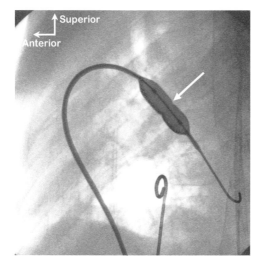

Fig. 27B

193

Pulmonary Arterial Angioplasty

Opposite: Pulmonary arterial angioplasty of stenotic branch pulmonary arteries.

> **Figure 28A** – Illustration showing uninflated angioplasty balloon in stenotic branch pulmonary artery

> **Figure 28B** – Angioplasty balloon inflated across stenosis relieving the obstruction

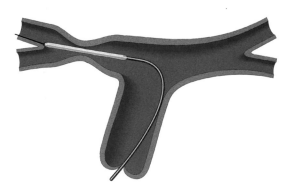

Fig. 28A

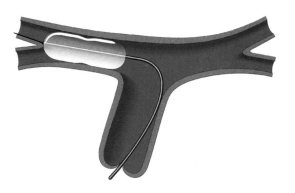

Fig. 28B

Aortic Coarctation Angioplasty

Angioplasty of recurrent coarctation following prior surgical repair has enjoyed fairly widespread success. However, angioplasty for native coarctation of the aorta is less well accepted because of a high rate of recurrence and the risk of late aneurysm formation. Therefore, angioplasty of native coarctation in the neonate is controversial. Sizing of the angioplasty balloon to be used for dilatation of a coarctation is dependent on the aortic isthmus size.

Opposite:

> **Figure 29A** – Angiogram showing lateral coarctation of the aorta
>
> C - coarctation, AAo - ascending aorta, DAo - descending aorta
>
> **Figure 29B** – Angioplasty balloon (indicated by arrow) inflated across coarctation site

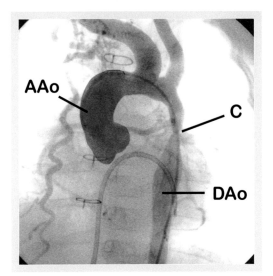

Fig. 29A

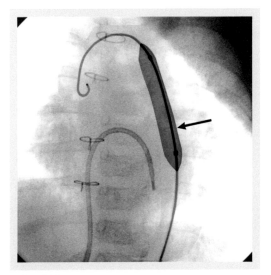

Fig. 29B

197

Illustrations of angioplasty for aortic coarctation are shown below and on the opposite page, demonstrating balloon and wire positioning.

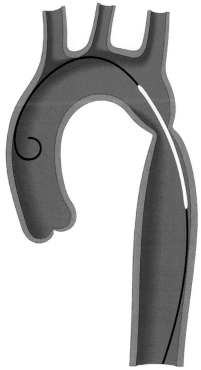

Fig. 30A

Above: Illustration shows uninflated angioplasty balloon positioned within coarctation of the descending aorta.

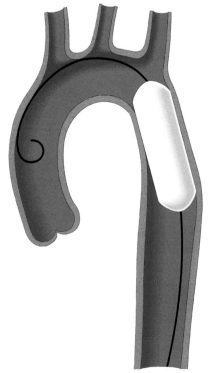

Fig. 30B

Above: Illustration shows angioplasty balloon inflated across coarctation site, stretching open the stenotic area.

INTRAVASCULAR STENTS

Balloon dilatable and self-expanding intravascular stents, developed for interventional radiologic indications, are broadly and frequently used in congenital cardiac catheterization procedures. Placement of intravascular stents for coarctation of the aorta have allowed improved hemodynamic results but do require slightly larger arterial sheaths for placement. Additionally, stents have been used in stenotic branch pulmonary arteries and pulmonary conduits where balloon angioplasty was ineffective (see page 202).

In general, stents placed in the pulmonary arterial tree for branch pulmonary artery stenosis have been somewhat more hemodynamically successful for the stenotic branch pulmonary artery lesion than angioplasty alone.

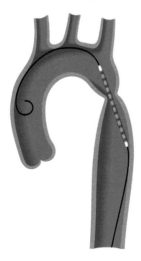

Above: Figure 31A – Stent mounted on an uninflated angioplasty balloon being passed through a coarctation

Opposite: Figure 31B – Expansion of the balloon and stent in the coarctation; **Figure 31C** - Deflation of the balloon leaving the stent fully expanded and opposed to the aortic wall

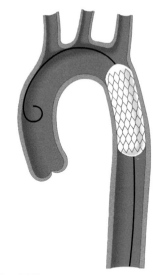

Fig. 31B

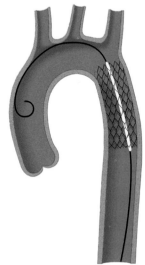

Fig. 31C

201

INTRAVASCULAR STENTS - continued

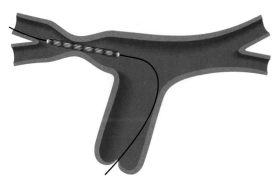

Above: Figure 32A – Stent mounted on an uninflated angioplasty balloon being passed through a stenotic pulmonary artery branch

Opposite: Figure 32B – Expansion of the balloon and stent in the branch pulmonary artery;

Figure 32C - Deflation of the balloon leaving the stent fully expanded and opposed to the branch pulmonary artery wall

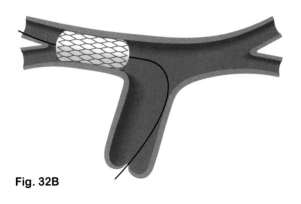

Fig. 32B

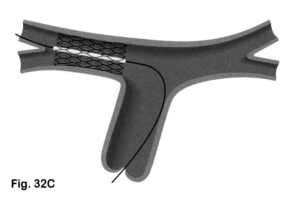

Fig. 32C

203

CHAPTER 5.
**PERCUTANEOUS VALVE INSERTION AND
REPAIR**

By D. Scott Lim, MD

Recently, rapid advances have occurred in the field of percutaneous transcatheter valve therapies, including valve repair and valve implantation. These novel options are undergoing investigation for failed pulmonary conduit valves, calcific aortic valve stenosis, and both degenerative and functional mitral regurgitation.

The following therapies are described here:

Percutaneous Pulmonary Valve Insertion

For patients with right ventricle-to-pulmonary artery conduit valves that have failed, either by stenosis or regurgitation, a transcatheter-delivered valve that has been mounted within a balloon-expandable stent is available. For the larger patient, this new valve insertion is a palliative procedure in that it extends the life of the right ventricle-to-pulmonary conduit. However, it is unlikely to be a permanent solution due to the high long-term failure rate of valves in this position subjected to the significant stress forces from other cardiac structures.

Due to the irregular nature of the native right ventricular outflow tract in patients with Tetralogy of Fallot, continued work is underway to design the appropriate transcatheter valve for this indication.

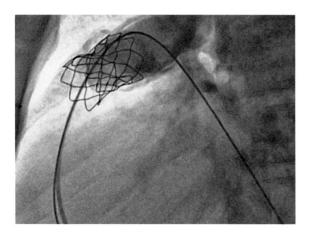

Above: Angiogram showing insertion of Melody valve into the right ventricular outflow tract

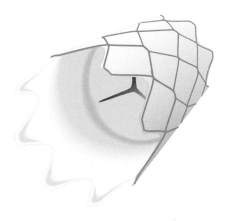

Above: Melody valve

Below: Melody valve insertion

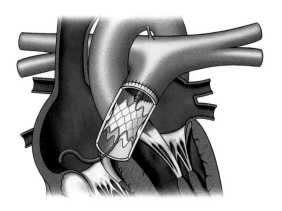

Transcatheter Aortic Valve Implantation

The rapid growth of implantation of transcatheter aortic valves has taken place primarily for patients with calcific aortic valve stenosis. Similar to the percutaneous pulmonary valve implants, the transcatheter aortic valves are bioprosthetic valves sewn within a balloon-expanded, or self-expanding stent.

The large delivery systems have been designed for either a retrograde transarterial or direct transapical approach. The utility of the direct transapical approach is that not all patients will have adequate femoral-iliac arteries to accommodate the 18-24 French delivery systems. For the balloon-expanded stent-valves, the ventricle is paced rapidly to limit cardiac output for careful device positioning. With the valve positioned too high or too low, paravalvar leaks or embolization may occur.

Opposite: Transcatheter aortic valve implantation insertion routes

Below: Edwards Sapien Transcatheter Heart Valve (THV)

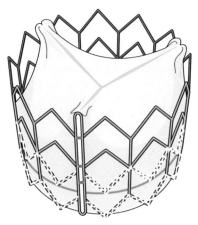

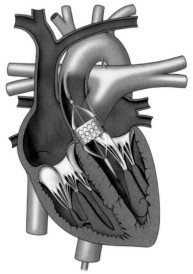

Transfemoral

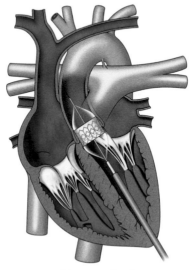

Transapical

Transcatheter Aortic Valve Implantation - continued

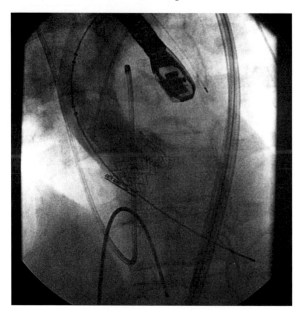

Above: Aortic angiography post transcatheter aortic valve implantation shows no paravalvar leak and valve is positioned well.

Percutaneous Mitral Valve Repair

A number of different types of devices to address mitral regurgitation are in various stages of design. However, to date only the MitraClip, a device designed to perform edge-to-edge repair of the mitral valve, has completed enrollment in randomized clinical trials. Other devices focusing on the mitral valve attempt to create an annuloplasty, but have not reached a randomized trial phase yet due to technical issues.

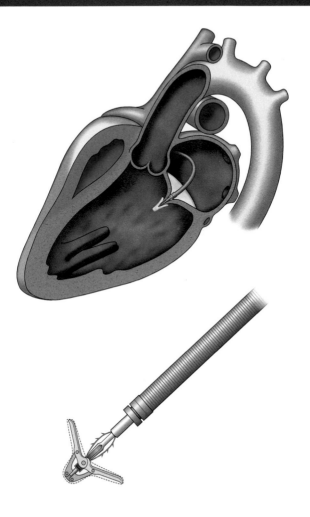

Above:

Top - Transcatheter mitral valve repair with the MitraClip is shown.

Bottom - detail of MitraClip

Percutaneous Mitral Valve Repair - continued

The MitraClip device is delivered by a transvenous, transseptal approach to the mitral valve, and is guided by transesophageal echocardiography. The device is implanted on the valve, grabbing the middle portions of the anterior and posterior mitral leaflets, creating a edge-to-edge repair, or a double-orifice mitral valve. It has been used with an excellent safety profile and reasonable efficacy results in the short and intermediate term. Both degenerative (prolapse and flail leaflets) and functional (annular dilation and mitral regurgitation secondary to cardiomyopathy) have been addressed by this novel technology.

Opposite:

Top - Angiogram showing transesophageal echocardiogram probe (TEE) and MitraClip (MC)

Bottom - Transesophageal echocardiogram demonstrates MitraClip in good position and no significant residual mitral regurgitation.

Mitral Valve - MV

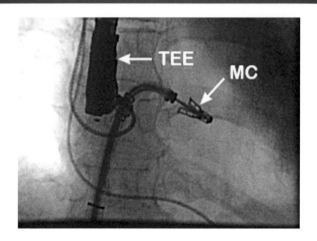

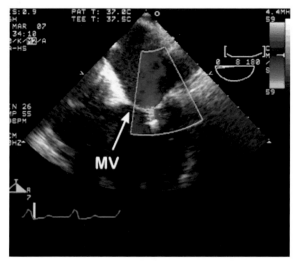

CHAPTER 6. **HYBRID INTERVENTIONS**

By D. Scott Lim, MD

HYBRID INTERVENTIONS

Historically, therapeutic procedures to address congenital heart disease were done as open surgical procedures in the operating room. With evolution of percutaneous therapies, some congenital lesions were amenable to the transcatheter approach and performed in the catheterization laboratory. Further evolution in the knowledge and technology have allowed innovative cardiologists and surgeons to combine their skill sets and approach difficult lesions through a combined, or hybrid interventional approach.

Hybrid interventions can either be a serial approach, where part of the complex lesion is addressed by percutaneous therapies, and part by open surgical approach, or by a more interdigitated approach where the transcatheter therapy is dependent upon open surgical access to the heart (see **Fig. 1, opposite**). In either approach, the key to a successful hybrid interventional program is close collaboration between cardiac and surgical physicians and staff.

VENTRICULAR SEPTAL DEFECT

While the majority of transcatheter device occlusions of ventricular septal defect (VSD) may be approached from an entirely percutaneous approach, certain patients and defects may be more amenable to a hybrid interventional approach. Patients that are too small for the percutaneous catheter delivery systems may be approached from an open sternotomy, and direct right ventricular access. The access point is determined by echocardiographic guidance, either transesophageal or epicardial, to aid in the most direct approach to the VSD. A purse-string suture is placed around the access needle in the right ventricular free wall, and then a wire is advanced across the VSD, over which the short delivery sheath is advanced to the left ventricle. The VSD occlusion device is then delivered to the defect and deployed, with the delivery sheath removed and the access point closed by the purse-string suture (**Fig. 2, opposite**).

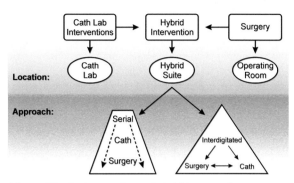

Above: Fig. 1. Approaches to hybrid intervention

Below: Fig. 2. Hybrid Ventricular Septal Defect occlusion

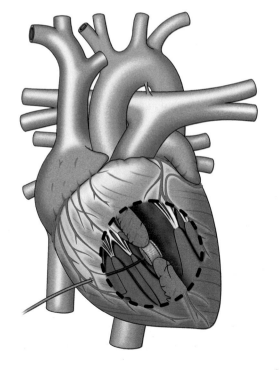

HYPOPLASTIC LEFT HEART SYNDROME

Palliation for Hypoplastic Left Heart Syndrome (HLHS) has frequently been either staged surgical palliation (Norwood, Glenn, and Fontan procedures) or cardiac transplantation. However, certain high risk patients with HLHS were not good candidates for staged surgical palliation, and while awaiting cardiac transplantation, investigators have looked into novel approaches to limit the pulmonary vascular injury from unprotected pulmonary blood flow. It is from these approaches that the hybrid palliation for HLHS has been derived.

The hybrid palliation for HLHS involves restricting pulmonary blood flow, insuring unimpeded systemic output, and unrestricted pulmonary venous return. The first step involves a surgical branch pulmonary artery banding, performed through an open sternotomy and without cardiopulmonary bypass. These pulmonary artery bands are to be removed at the second stage palliation.

The second step creates unimpeded systemic cardiac output via the ductus arteriosus. Either self-expanding or balloon-expanded stents are placed in the ductus to insure its continued patency once prostaglandin E1 is discontinued. With this step, it is extremely important to cover the entire ductus with stent, as any residual ductal tissue will contract producing significant obstruction to systemic outflow. The stent may be delivered either from a transvenous approach, or from a direct insertion into the main pulmonary artery.

The final step, is to relieve any obstruction to pulmonary venous return at the atrial septum. This usually involves a balloon septostomy. However in patients with HLHS, the atrial septum may be unusually thick, and the atrial septal defect in an unusually superior position, making a dynamic balloon septostomy difficult. However, performing a static balloon dilation of the septum frequently doesn't

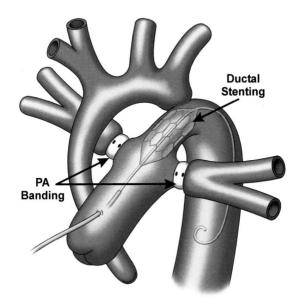

Figure 3. Hybrid palliation of Hypoplastic Left Heart Syndrome (PA - pulmonary arteries)

tear a large enough opening. Therefore, some operators have chosen to place a stent across the atrial communication.

Patients returning for the second stage palliation of HLHS following first stage hybrid palliation will require a "comprehensive" surgery – debanding of the branch pulmonary arteries, resection of the stented ductus arteriosus and reconstruction of the neo-aortic outflow, atrial septectomy, and construction of the cavo-pulmonary anastomosis. Investigators at a few sites have also looked at using the "comprehensive" second stage palliation to set up the 3rd stage to be a transcatheter Fontan completion.

219

TRANSCATHETER AORTIC VALVE IMPLANTATION

For patients at increased surgical risk for the standard surgical aortic valve replacement, transcatheter aortic valve implantation has evolved and is currently in clinical trials. These novel valves are tissue valves sewed within either a self-expanding or balloon-expanded stent.

Due to the large caliber of the delivery sheaths (18 – 26 French) and the frequent concomitant presence of peripheral artery disease, not all patients will be served by a percutaneous transfemoral approach (see page 209). Therefore, a hybrid transapical approach has evolved. A limited left-sided thoracotomy is performed gaining access to the left ventricular apex, through which the large delivery sheath is directly inserted into the left ventricle. Following valve delivery, the sheath is removed and the apical insertion site is closed by purse string sutures.

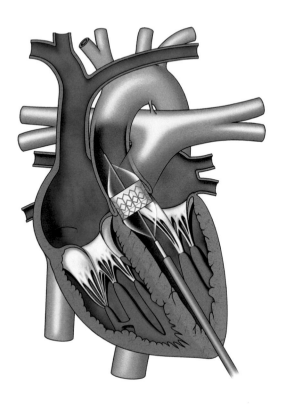

Figure 4. Transapical approach to the transcatheter aortic valve implantation

CHAPTER 7.
CONGENITAL HEART SURGERIES

By Marshall L. Jacobs, MD and Luca A. Vricella, MD

Absent Pulmonary Valve Repair

Absent Pulmonary Valve Syndrome is a very rare variant of tetralogy of Fallot. The objectives of surgical repair are relief of right ventricular outflow tract obstruction, elimination of shunting at the ventricular level, and reduction of compression of the central airways by the aneurysmal pulmonary arteries. The ventricular septal defect is closed with a patch. The right ventricular outflow tract may be augmented with a transannular patch, or alternatively may be reconstructed by insertion of a homograft or bioprosthetic pulmonary valve (light blue in the illustrations **opposite**). As the pulmonary arteries are often significantly dilated in this defect, a reduction arterioplasty (anterior, or both anterior and posterior) may be performed at the same time.

Aneurysmal dilatation of the main and branch pulmonary arteries, compressing the central airways, may result in the development of severe bronchomalacia. As an alternative to, or in conjunction with reduction arterioplasty, the pulmonary bifurcation may be brought anterior to the ascending aorta (LeCompte maneuver) as a means of eliminating airway compression.

Options for valve replacement include aortic or pulmonary homografts or other bioprosthetic valved conduits, such as bovine internal jugular vein (Contegra®) or porcine bioprostheses (Hancock®) among others.

In the tetralogy variant with absent pulmonary valve, a patent ductus arteriosus is an extremely rare finding. Absent pulmonary valve may co-exist with intact ventricular septum however, in which case a patent ductus is almost always present.

Opposite: Upper Left - External view of heart, with internal ventricular septal defect indicated by dashed oval; **Upper Right** - Trunk of the pulmonary artery is excised (right arrow) and the right ventricular outflow tract is widened (left arrow); **Middle Left** - Opening in pulmonary artery branches is narrowed to receive prosthetic valve; **Middle Right** - A prosthetic valved conduit (light blue) is attached to the pulmonary artery branches and the right ventricle; **Bottom** – The ventricular septal defect is patched (pink oval).

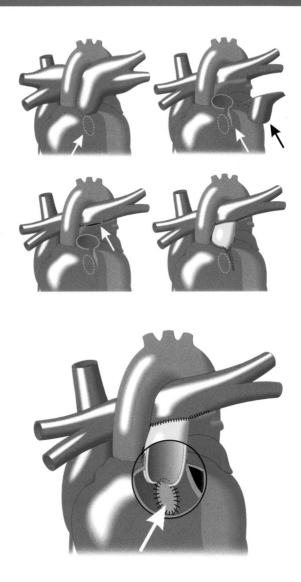

The objective of repair is to establish antegrade flow into the entire coronary artery system with oxygenated blood from the aorta. Historically, in the face of adequate intercoronary collaterals, the condition was treated by ligation of the anomalous pulmonary artery origin of the left coronary artery. Contemporary management is aimed at establishment of a two coronary artery system.

There are various ways in which this can be accomplished. Whenever possible, the left coronary artery is reimplanted into the aorta by transposing the ostium of the coronary artery with a surrounding button of tissue from the pulmonary artery to the aorta. Alternatively, aortic flow may be directed to the anomalous left coronary artery through a surgically created aorto-pulmonary window via a baffle to the coronary ostium within the pulmonary artery (Takeuchi procedure).[1]

The anomaly may present with severe left ventricular dysfunction and varying degrees of mitral valve regurgitation. While both of these phenomena generally improve over time after successful repair, some neonates and infants undergoing repair of this anomaly may also require surgical correction of the associated severe mitral regurgitation and are at high risk for requiring ventricular assistance with extra-corporeal membranous oxygenation in the postoperative period.

Opposite:

> **Top:** Uncorrected anomalous left coronary artery (PA - pulmonary artery, AO - Aorta)

> **Middle:** Anomalous left coronary artery with button of tissue is detached from pulmonary artery

> **Bottom:** Left coronary artery with button of tissue is sutured to the Aorta

---

[1] See also the Takeuchi Procedure, page 292.

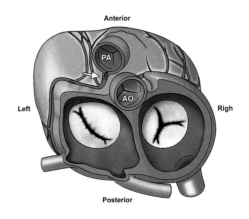

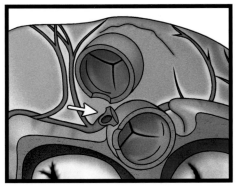

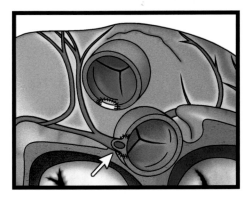

The objectives of the operation are to create an unobstructed pathway or connection of all of the pulmonary veins to the left atrium, and the elimination of any left-to-right or right-to-left shunts. The surgical repair of partial anomalous pulmonary venous return involves either direct anastomosis of the anomalously draining vein(s) to the left atrium and closure of any connection with the systemic venous system or the construction of a baffle to direct blood from the anomalous vein to the left atrium.

The rerouting baffle (in light blue, opposite) is constructed with autologous pericardium or expanded polytetrafluorethylene (ePTFE). If no ASD is present, a communication is surgically created.

Occasionally, partial anomalous pulmonary venous connection to the right superior vena cava is associated with a high (sinus venosus) type of inter-atrial communication (ASD). This anomaly may be treated by baffling of the pulmonary venous return through the inter-atrial communication to the left atrium and patch enlargement of the junction of the superior vena cava (SVC) with the right atrium. Alternatively, the SVC may be transected above the entrance of the anomalously connected pulmonary vein(s) and then anastomosed to the right atrial appendage. The inter-atrial baffle is also constructed. This operation (Warden procedure - not shown) may be more likely to preserve the blood supply and integrity of the sinoatrial node.

Opposite:

(top) The anomalous right upper pulmonary vein entering the superior vena cava is baffled over to the left atrium via the sinus venosus atrial septal defect. (Abbreviations: RLPV - right lower pulmonary vein, RUPV - right upper pulmonary vein, LUPV - left upper pulmonary vein, LLPV - left lower pulmonary vein, SVC - superior vena cava)

(bottom) Note patch on superior vena cava (shown in light blue), which allows unobstructed superior vena caval return.

230

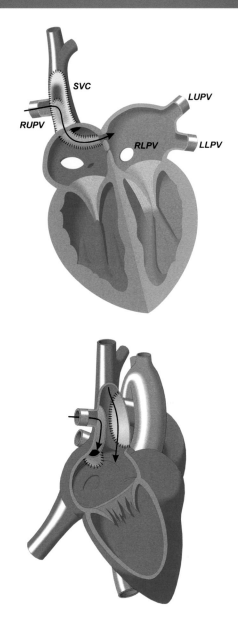

The illustrations show the repair of a common type of total anomalous pulmonary venous connection (supra-cardiac). The general principle of creating a wide anastomosis between the confluence of the pulmonary veins and the left atrium applies in the setting of other anatomic types as well (infra-cardiac and cardiac total anomalous pulmonary venous connection).

The left atrium and the confluence of pulmonary veins are opened and sutured together. Notice (in **Figure 2**, opposite) that the vertical vein that connects the pulmonary venous confluence to the innominate vein is ligated and may be divided to minimize tension on the anastomosis of the pulmonary vein confluence to the left atrium.

The atrial septal defect (3 in **Figure 2,** opposite) is closed with a patch to augment the often small left atrium. The ductus arteriosus is routinely ligated (not shown in the illustration).

Opposite:

> **Figure 1** - Internal view of a heart with total anomalous pulmonary venous return. Note the left-sided vertical vein draining the pulmonary venous confluence to the innominate vein (IV). An incision is made in the posterior wall of the left atrium (indicated by lower arrow).

> **Figure 2:**

>> **1** - The vertical vein draining the anomalous pulmonary venous confluence is ligated and divided.

>> **2** - The anomalous pulmonary venous confluence and left atrium are sutured together, creating a passage between pulmonary veins and left atrium.

>> **3** - The atrial septal defect is closed by a patch (patch shown in pink).

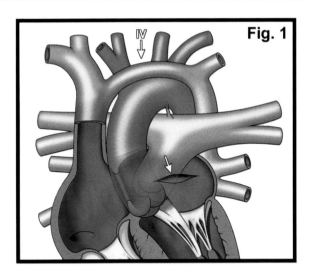

Fig. 1

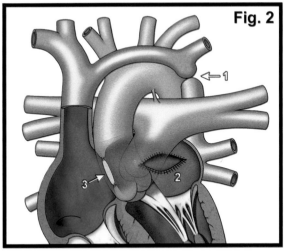

Fig. 2

233

Aortopulmonary Window Repair

The connection (window) between the aorta and pulmonary artery is closed with a patch made of pericardium or synthetic material. The communication may be approached from within the pulmonary artery or through the aorta. Care must be exercised to avoid distortion of a coronary artery origin, or narrowing of the proximal portion of a branch pulmonary artery (usually the right). This patch (pink oval in the illustration) is sutured into place and the incision in either of the two vessels through which the patch was introduced is closed with sutures.

Opposite:

> **Upper Left** - Internal view of heart, showing a common position of the aortopulmonary window
>
> **Upper Right** - Close-up of the aortopulmonary window
>
> **Lower Left** - The aortopulmonary window is closed with a patch (pink oval).
>
> **Lower Right** - The patch is sutured into place.

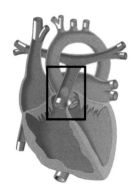
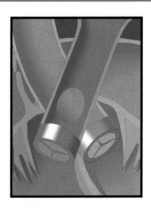
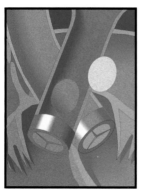
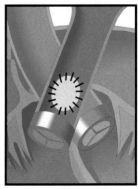

235

Arterial Switch Operation (Jatene)

This operation is performed to treat infants with *d*-transposition of the great arteries. For the most common form of transposition, with intact ventricular septum, the arterial switch operation is generally performed within the first few weeks of life. Surgery may be performed at that time, or later in infancy, if a hemodynamically significant ventricular septal defect is present.

The "switch" operation involves transection of both the aorta and the main pulmonary artery and then connection of the distal ascending aorta to the proximal main pulmonary artery (and thus the left ventricle), and connection of the pulmonary artery confluence to the proximal aorta (and thus the right ventricle). The critical feature of the operation is the transfer of each coronary artery origin, together with a surrounding button or arterial wall, from the native aorta to the "neo-aorta."

Commonly, in performing the arterial switch procedure the surgeon will bring the confluence of the pulmonary arteries in front of the reconstructed aorta (the LeCompte maneuver) so that the left and right branch pulmonary arteries straddle the ascending aorta in their posterior course to the lungs. If the pulmonary arteries are not mobilized adequately, branch pulmonary artery stenosis can result.

The degree of difficulty associated with the transfer and reimplantation of the coronary arteries is variable, depending upon the specific anatomy of the origins and course of the principle coronary branches. Any atrial communication (ASD) is closed (**2** in illustrations opposite) and the patent ductus arteriosus (PDA - **1** in illustrations opposite) is divided.

Opposite: Top – Arterial switch operation, including closure of PDA (**1**) and ASD (**2**). Note that the pulmonary bifurcation is now relocated in front of the aorta (LeCompte maneuver); **Bottom, left** - Transfer of the coronary arteries to the pulmonary root (neo-aorta); **Bottom, right** - *d*-Transposition of the great arteries, before surgery (**1** – PDA, **2** – ASD, **3** – transposition) of PDA (**1**) and ASD (**2**).

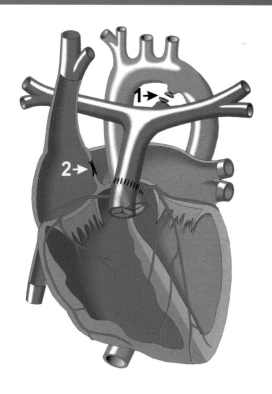

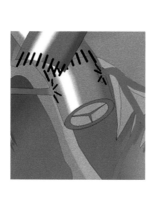

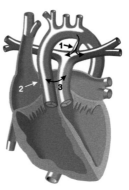

237

The simplest forms of atrial septal defect (ostium secundum type and patent foramen ovale) may be closed using a patch or by direct suture during open-heart surgery, or through the use of a trans-catheter device, such as a septal occluder.[1]

Minimally invasive surgical approaches involve special instruments that are inserted into 3 or 4 small incisions or "ports" in the chest.

During surgical correction, small defects may be closed with a running suture. Larger holes should be closed with a patch of pericardium (the membrane that covers the heart) or of a synthetic material such as Dacron or expanded polytetrafluorethylene (ePTFE).

Opposite:

A large secundum-type atrial septal defect is repaired by suturing a patch (pink oval) to the edges of the defect.

---

[1]See page 172*ff* for occlusion of atrial septal defects.

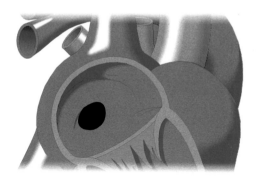

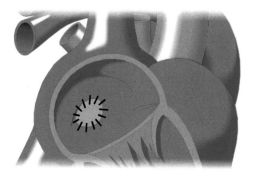

The Mustard Repair and Senning Atrial Switch Procedures for *d*-transposition of the great arteries were commonly performed prior to the advent of successful anatomic repair of transposition of the great arteries (TGA) by means of the arterial switch procedure. The indications for these "atrial switch" operations are somewhat limited today. The Mustard and Senning procedures, designed in the early era of congenital heart surgery, both direct the oxygen-rich blood entering the heart from the pulmonary veins to the aorta via the right ventricle and the deoxygenated blood entering the heart from the vena cava to the pulmonary artery via the left ventricle.

In the Mustard Repair (**opposite**), this is achieved by removing the atrial septum and constructing a baffle made of pericardium or prosthetic material that channels blood from the vena cava to the left ventricle via the mitral valve. The blood entering the heart from the pulmonary veins is directed by this baffle to enter the right ventricle through the tricuspid valve.

In the physiologically similar procedure known as the Senning Procedure (not shown), the baffle is constructed using a flap of autologous atrial tissue rather than from pericardium. The use of the Senning and Mustard procedures today is largely limited to patients with *l*-transposition of the great arteries (congenitally corrected transposition of the great arteries) in whom the Double Switch Procedure is used (Atrial and Arterial Switches). These procedures also have a limited role in the management of patients with simple transposition of the great arteries who present beyond the newborn period.

Opposite: Mustard Repair

> **Top** - View of heart after Mustard Repair showing circulation; **Bottom Left** - Oxygen-rich blood (red arrows) from the pulmonary veins is directed over the baffle and through the tricuspid valve into the right ventricle and to the aorta; **Bottom Right** - Oxygen-poor blue arrows behind the baffle) from the superior and inferior venae cavae is directed through the mitral valve into the left ventricle, and out the pulmonary artery.

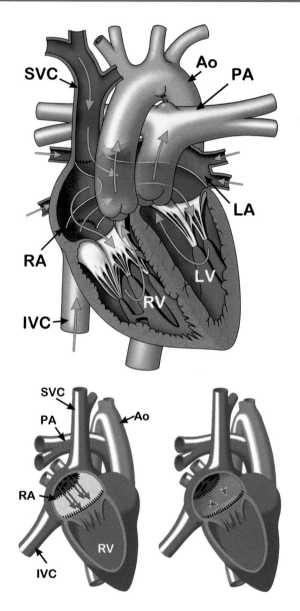

241

In repair of atrioventricular septal defect (AVSD), the deficiencies of the septa dividing the atria and ventricles (**Figures 1** and **3**) must be addressed. Repair of complete AVSD (or complete common atrioventricular canal defect) may be accomplished with a single patch (as shown in **Figure 2**), usually made of pericardium or Dacron, or with two separate patches; one to complete the atrial septum and one to complete the ventricular septum. In addition, two separate atrioventricular valves must be fashioned from the tissue of the common atrioventricular valve. The zone of apposition ("cleft") between superior and inferior elements of the septal leaflet of the new left-sided valve is usually, but not always, approximated with sutures (left arrow in **Figure 4**).

Opposite:

> **Figure 1** - Internal view of heart showing atrioventricular septal defect, complete (note: aorta and pulmonary artery are not shown)

> **Figure 2** - A single patch (pink, indicated by arrow) is sutured into place to separate the atria, ventricles, and left and right atrioventricular valves.

> **Figure 3** - Superior view of heart showing the common atrioventricular valve (the arrow points to the zone of apposition that will become the "cleft" of the left atrioventricular valve).

> **Figure 4** - Superior view is shown of the patch (pink, indicated by right arrow), which separates the atria, ventricles (not visible), and left and right sided valves. The "cleft" in the left-sided valve has been closed (left arrow).

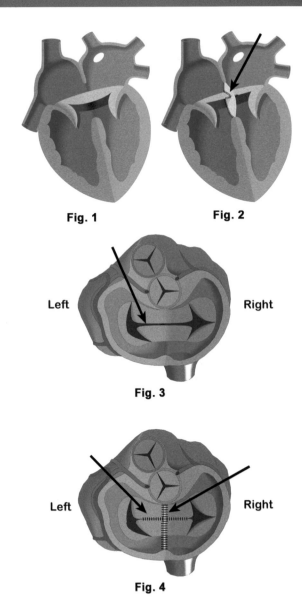

Fig. 1

Fig. 2

Left

Right

Fig. 3

Left

Right

Fig. 4

243

In the repair of a partial atrioventricular septal defect (also referred to as primum atrial septal defect), the "cleft" in the left atrioventricular valve is repaired with simple sutures. The primum atrial septal defect is closed by suturing a patch (pink in the illustration) to the edges of the defect and to the fibrous tissue on the crest of the interventricular septum.

Opposite:

> **Upper Left** - Internal view of heart from the left anterior- oblique position showing partial atrioventricular septal defect

> **Upper Right** - Close-up showing the "cleft" between the superior and inferior septal elements of the left atrioventricular valve and low-lying atrial septal defect (ASD, primum atrial component)

> **Lower Left** - Repair of left-sided valve by suturing of cleft (arrow)

> **Lower Right** - Repair of atrial septal defect with patch (shown in pink, indicated by arrow)

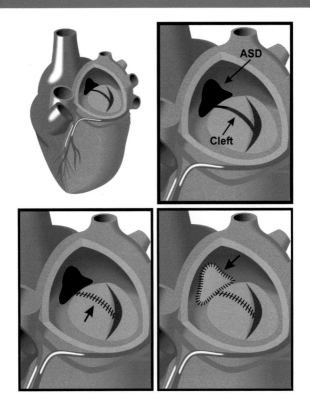

245

The Modified Blalock-Taussig Shunt is designed to provide a calibrated amount of pulmonary blood flow. It is used in two ventricle defects in which there is insufficient pulmonary blood flow or in functionally univentricular heart anomalies in which pulmonary blood flow must be restricted in order to protect the pulmonary vascular bed for planned Fontan circulation.

This palliative procedure involves interposing a graft (expanded polytetrafluorethylene (ePTFE) or cryopreserved homograft vein) between the innominate or subclavian artery and the right or left pulmonary artery. As a rule, the shunt is placed on the side opposite the aortic arch.

Some older patients may have had a "classic" Blalock-Taussig Shunt performed. This involved transecting the subclavian artery and directly anastamosing it in an end-to-side fashion to either left or right pulmonary arteries. The classic Blalock-Taussig Shunt is not typically performed today.

The procedure was originally performed through a right or left thoracotomy, depending on the neonate's particular anatomy. In more recent times, the procedure is accomplished by many surgeons via a median sternotomy. An anterior approach allows the surgeon to ligate the arterial duct and have access to cardio-pulmonary bypass in case of cardio-respiratory instability. A sternotomy approach allows for a shorter shunt which can be placed more centrally, thus reducing the likelihood of compromise of blood flow to the right or left upper lobe arterial branches. It allows for further palliation or deferred complete repair to be performed through one incision. Resternotomy, of course, is necessary at the time of definitive repair. Typical shunt sizes are 3.0, 3.5 and 4.0 mm, and are chosen according to operative weight.

Opposite:

> **Top** - Modified Blalock-Taussig Shunt Procedure

> **Bottom right** - Tricuspid atresia after the Modified Blalock-Taussig Shunt

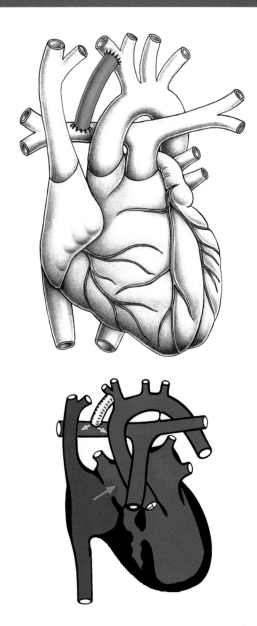

247

Historically, a number of different operative techniques have been used to treat aortic coarctation. These include: 1) Coarctation excision with end-to-end anastomosis, 2) patch enlargement of the narrowed aortic segment, 3) subclavian flap repair (see **page 250**), or 4) excision with extended end-to-end anastomosis. In cases of transverse aortic arch hypoplasia with coarctation, coarctation excision with end-to-end anastomosis and reverse subclavian flap repair may be used in combination.

In neonates, balloon angioplasty is generally avoided and surgical repair is favored. In older patients, balloon angioplasty with or without stent placement is sometimes used. A stent (expandable rigid endovascular tube) may be inserted by means of a catheterization procedure to widen the affected part of the aorta and keep it open (see **page 200**).

In the illustrations on the **opposite** page, the coarctation is surgically repaired by excision of the obstructing portion of the descending aorta and suturing together the resulting ends (an "end-to-end" repair, upper arrow on bottom illustration).

Notice that, as is usual in coarctation of the aorta, the narrowing is directly opposite the patent ductus arteriosus (PDA).

In the case shown here, the patent ductus arteriosus is divided and its aortic end is removed with the constricted section of the aorta. The pulmonary end is ligated.

Opposite: Excision with End-to-End Anastamosis

>   **Figure 1** - Coarctation of the aorta (COA), patent ductus arteriosus (PDA)

>   **Figure 2** - Removal of coarctation and patent ductus arteriosus

>   **Figure 3** - Anastomosis of the aorta on either side of the removed coarctation (upper arrow) and closure of ductal remnant on pulmonary artery (lower arrow)

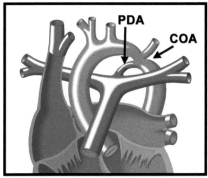

Fig. 1

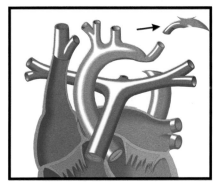

Fig. 2

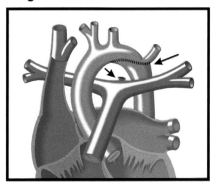

Fig. 3

Another operation for coarctation of the aorta is known as the Subclavian Flap Angioplasty. This involves opening up the aorta in the region of the coarctation and the subclavian artery, then folding down the opened subclavian artery section over the area of the coarctation and suturing it to the aorta as a patch.

This accomplishes effective augmentation of the aortic arch, without resection of the coarctation. It avoids the need for a circumferential suture line and augments the narrow section of aorta using viable arterial tissue. This procedure is a viable option in neonates and infants, in whom interruption of the left subclavian artery is usually well-tolerated without major consequences.

Opposite:

> **Figure 1** - Coarctation of the aorta (COA), patent ductus arteriosus (PDA), subclavian artery (SCA)

> **Figure 2** - Incisions made to aorta and lower subclavian artery, which is opened as a flap, ductus arteriosus is ligated

> **Figure 3** - Anastomosed subclavian flap and aorta, ligation of subclavian artery

> **Figure 4** (upper right) - Close-up of anastomosis of subclavian flap (SCAF) to aorta

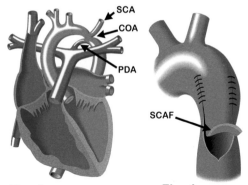

Fig. 1

Fig. 4

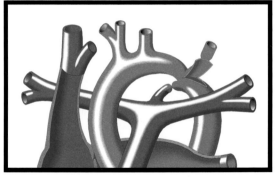

Fig. 2

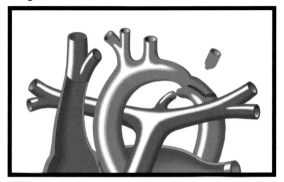

Fig. 3

251

This procedure provides unobstructed systemic outflow in some functionally univentricular hearts by anastamosing the divided proximal main pulmonary artery to the ascending aorta. The aorta and pulmonary artery are sutured together above their respective valves in this procedure (see **opposite**, below). Pulmonary blood flow is generally provided by a modified Blalock-Taussig Shunt from a branch of the aorta to one of the branches of the pulmonary artery. Homograft material (a patch made of human tissue that has been cryopreserved) or autologous pericardium is used to augment the area where the ascending aorta is joined to both pulmonary and aortic roots. Alternately, the pulmonary artery can be connected directly to the ascending aorta in an end-to-side fashion, avoiding use of a patch.

Typically, a Damus-Kaye-Stansel (DKS) procedure is chosen when a functionally univentricular heart has obstruction to flow into the aorta (systemic circulation) and unrestricted flow into the lungs. The procedure, in combination with a shunt, provides relief of systemic ventricular outflow obstruction at the same time as it regulates pulmonary blood flow.

Opposite:

Top: Damus-Kaye-Stansel Procedure with right Modified Blalock-Taussig Shunt

1. Modified Blalock-Taussig Shunt
2. Pulmonary homograft
3. Pulmonary artery
4. Aorta

Bottom: Suturing together of the aorta and pulmonary artery above the valve opening

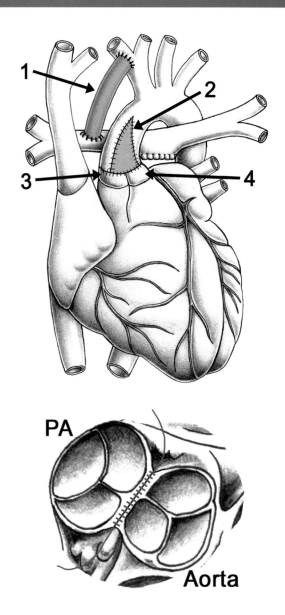

253

In Double Outlet Right Ventricle (DORV) with sub-aortic ventricular septal defect (VSD), intraventricular repair can generally be accomplished by baffling the left ventricular outflow via the VSD to the aorta. When the morphology is not favorable for an intraventricular repair, or in the case of significant pulmonary stenosis, then the pulmonary valve may be sacrificed in order to gain sufficient space to place an intraventricular baffle. Right ventricle to pulmonary artery continuity is then established by an extracardiac conduit, the so-called Rastelli operation (illustrated **opposite**).

If the aorta is remote from the ventricular septal defect (DORV with subpulmonary VSD, "transposition type"), it may be practical to baffle the left ventricular output to the aorta only when there is sufficient distance between the tricuspid annulus and the pulmonary valve (generally a distance equal to or greater than the size of the aortic annulus). This is the Kawashima procedure.

When the tricuspid-pulmonary distance is inadequate, such cases would in the past be amenable to a modification of the Damus-Kaye-Stansel procedure (see **page 252**). Here, the proximal pulmonary artery-to-aortic amalgamation provides the outflow to the aorta, the left ventricle is baffled to the pulmonary valve, and a conduit is interposed between the right ventricle and the pulmonary arteries. Contemporary management consists of baffling the left ventricle to the pulmonary valve and performing an arterial switch procedure (see **page 236**).

In double outlet right ventricle associated with hypoplasia of the right or left heart, or when the VSD cannot be committed to the aorta, single ventricular surgical palliation is an option, eventually leading to the Fontan Procedure (see **page 260**).

Opposite: Top Left - Double outlet right ventricle with doubly committed ventricular septal defect (VSD); **Top Right** - The main pulmonary artery is transected and oversewn proximally. A baffle, or VSD patch, is inserted (pink), directing left ventricular output through the VSD to the aorta; **Bottom** - Placement of valved conduit (light blue) to route systemic venous blood from the right ventricle to the pulmonary arteries

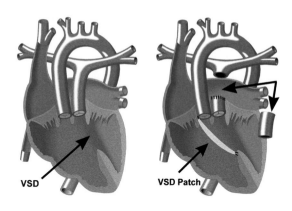

VSD

VSD Patch

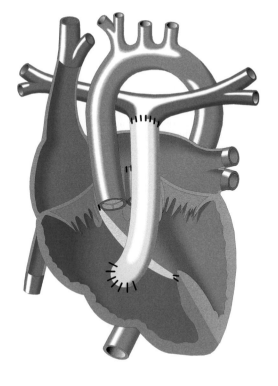

255

Surgery in the neonatal period may be necessary in cases of Ebstein's anomaly in which tricuspid valve regurgitation is severe and results in cyanosis and poor perfusion. Tricuspid valve repair in the neonatal period can be very challenging. Alternatives to bi-ventricular repair include patch closure of the tricuspid valve and conversion to single ventricle physiology (Starnes Procedure) and cardiac transplantation.

In older patients, tricuspid valve repair is frequently possible, as an alternative to tricuspid valve replacement. Ebstein's anomaly repair techniques (Danielson and Carpentier) aim to reduce the size of the tricuspid valve annulus and utilize the available functional leaflet tissue (anterior leaflet, generally) in order to create a competent valve. Repair frequently includes plication of the atrialized portion of the right ventricle.

Opposite: Carpentier's Procedure

> **Figure 1** - Internal view from above of a heart with Ebstein's anomaly
>
> > TV - tricuspid valve, MV- mitral valve
> > LV - left ventricle, RV - right ventricle
> > AO - aorta, PA - pulmonary artery
>
> **Figure 2** - The anterior leaflet of the tricuspid valve is mobilized (arrow).
>
> **Figure 3** - Vertical plication of the atrialized portion of the right ventricle (arrow)
>
> **Figure 4** - Anterior leaflet of tricuspid valve is advanced across the plicated area and reduces the size of the valve orifice (arrow).
>
> **Figure 5** - Annular ring (arrow) is sutured into place to strengthen the tricuspid valve.

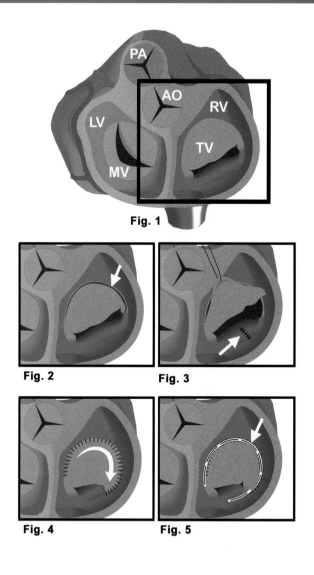

Fig. 1

Fig. 2

Fig. 3

Fig. 4

Fig. 5

257

Some modification of the Fontan/Kreutzer Procedure is the definitive therapy for functionally univentricular hearts. The general principle involves separation of the systemic and pulmonary circulations, arranging them in series without the contribution of a sub-pulmonary ventricle. Venous blood flows directly to the lungs, then returning to the systemic ventricle.

The illustration opposite depicts an atrio-pulmonary connection – an early or "classic" form of the Fontan procedure, in which the right atrial appendage was anastamosed to the main pulmonary artery to direct blood flow from the superior and inferior vena cavae into the pulmonary artery. This procedure is no longer performed because of the subsequent dilation of the right atrium resulting in severe atrial dysrhythmias and atrial thrombi (see **pages 260-261** for the current forms of the Fontan procedure, including extracardiac and lateral tunnel total cavopulmonary connections).

Opposite:

      Top - Internal view of tricuspid atresia after the classic Fontan/Kreutzer Procedure

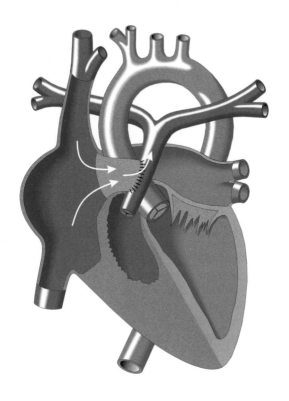

The total cavopulmonary connection (modified Fontan Procedure) is generally performed after a hemi-Fontan or bidirectional Glenn anastomosis. If the pulmonary vascular resistance is sufficiently low, separation of the arterial and venous circulations is completed with the modified Fontan repair. In this procedure, a pathway (or tunnel) is fashioned to connect the inferior vena cava to the pulmonary artery. This tunnel may be constructed either inside or outside of the heart (lateral atrial tunnel or extra-cardiac conduit Fontan, respectively). After this procedure, the patient's oxygen saturations are near normal as the systemic and pulmonary venous circulations are now separated.

A small opening (fenestration) in the venous pathway (indicated by arrows in the illustrations **opposite**) may be created to provide a pop-off for venous blood to the left side, if right-sided pressures are high. This will preserve cardiac output at the expense of some degree of desaturation. When no longer required, the fenestration may close spontaneously or may be closed in the cardiac catheterization laboratory, without the need for another surgical procedure.[1]

Opposite:

> **Top** - Extra-cardiac Conduit Fontan procedure. The connecting tunnel is usually made of expanded polytetrafluoroethylene (ePTFE). (Arrow indicates site of fenestration.)

> **Bottom** - Lateral atrial tunnel Fontan procedure. (Arrow indicates site of fenestration and direction of blood flow.)

---

[1] See page 182*f* for transcatheter closure of a Fontan fenestration.

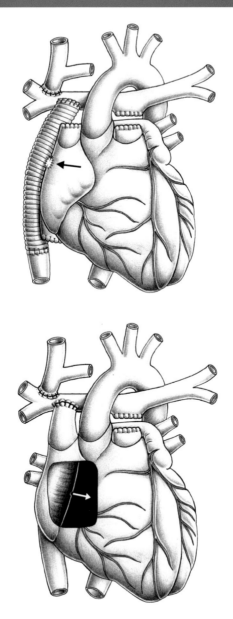

Glenn Shunt Procedure (Bidirectional)

The bidirectional Glenn shunt (BDG) is a superior cavopulmonary anastomosis. It is often an intermediate step towards the complete separation of the pulmonary and systemic circulations in patients with functionally univentricular hearts (e.g. tricuspid atresia). Complete separation is achieved with the Fontan procedure, or Total Cavo-Pulmonary Connection.

Typically, the Glenn Procedure is the second procedure in single ventricle palliation and is performed on children between 4 and 9 months of life. Most children with functionally univentricular hearts will have undergone surgical palliation in the neonatal period, involving the calibration of the pulmonary blood flow by a direct systemic-to-pulmonary artery shunt (most often a modified Blalock-Taussig shunt) or by banding of the pulmonary artery. After maturation of the pulmonary vasculature, they may undergo the superior cavopulmonary anastomosis (BDG), which provides adequate pulmonary bloodflow but reduces the volume work of the "single ventricle."

In the Glenn procedure, the Blalock-Taussig shunt (if present) is ligated or clamped and disconnected from the pulmonary artery. Other sources of pulmonary blood flow, such as antegrade flow through a stenotic pulmonary valve or banded pulmonary artery are generally eliminated as well. The divided superior vena cava is connected to the right pulmonary artery, which remains in continuity with the left pulmonary artery. This allows deoxygenated blood from the head and neck to flow directly into the pulmonary arteries. In addition, the azygous vein is generally ligated. The pulmonary-to-systemic blood flow ratio (Qp/Qs) is approximately 0.6:1 after the superior cavopulmonary anastomosis, but varies somewhat with age and size of the patient.

Opposite:

> **Top** - Bidirectional Glenn shunt procedure

> **Bottom** - Blood flow in tricuspid atresia after the bidirectional Glenn shunt procedure

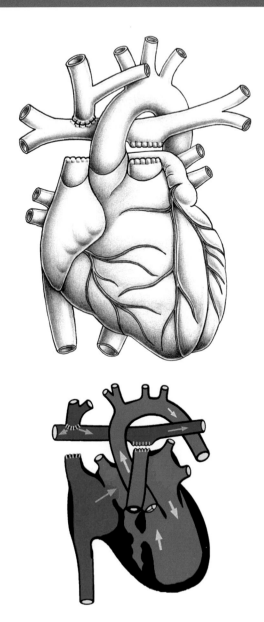

Hemi-Fontan Procedure

The hemi-Fontan procedure is a type of superior cavopulmonary anastomosis that is intended to simplify the eventual completion of the Fontan circulation. In this procedure, the superior vena cava is associated with the pulmonary arteries, directing the venous flow from the upper body to the lungs. A patch or dam of either homograft material or polytetrafluoroethylene (PTFE) (blue in diagram **opposite**, top) is placed between the superior vena cava and the right atrium in order to divert upper body systemic return into the pulmonary artery.

An additional patch is used to augment the amalgamation of the superior vena cava with the pulmonary arteries and to address any stenosis or distortion in the branch pulmonary arteries. This patch, shown in red on the illustration (**opposite**, bottom), may be homograft or pericardium. Some surgeons use a single large patch of homograft for both the atrial dam and the pulmonary artery patch.

A hemi-Fontan, rather than a Bi-Directional Glenn, is mainly utilized when the surgeon plans a lateral tunnel (as opposed to an extra-cardiac conduit) to eventually accomplish completion of the total cavopulmonary connection. At the time of the completion Fontan procedure, the dam closing the junction of the superior vena cava with the right atrium is excised, and the lateral atrial tunnel is constructed.

Below: Hypoplastic left heart syndrome after the Hemi-Fontan Procedure

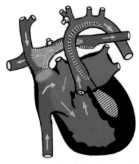

Opposite: Top – Homograft baffle (blue); **Bottom** – Patch (red) augmentation of amalgamation of SVC and pulmonary arteries.

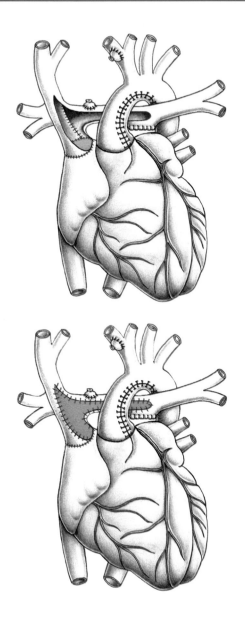

265

The various types of aortic arch interruption are described on **page 74**. The goals of surgical correction are establishment of unobstructed continuity between ascending and descending aorta and repair of associated defects (most commonly ventricular septal defect and/or atrial septal defect). The patent ductus arteriosus is also ligated and divided as part of the procedure (2, 3 in upper right illustration).

The distal portion of the aorta is mobilized and anastomosed to the aorta proximal to the interruption, often in an end-to-side fashion (4 in bottom illustration). The anastomosis may consist entirely of native arterial tissue, or alternatively may be augmented with a homograft or autograft vascular patch. Also, the ventricular septal defect (VSD) is closed (5) with a patch of synthetic material such as Dacron or expanded polytetrafluoroethylene (ePTFE).

An alternative to definitive repair of the arch and associated defects in a single operation is a two-stage approach. This consists of arch reconstruction and placement of a pulmonary artery band as a first stage palliation. VSD closure or repair of other defects is deferred to a later time. The pulmonary artery band is removed during the second stage procedure.

Opposite:

> **Top Left** - Internal view of a heart with interrupted aortic arch, Type B

> **Top Right -**
>> 1 - An incision is made to open up the ascending aorta section (aortotomy) to allow anastomosis to the descending aorta section.
>> 2 - The patent ductus arteriosus is removed.
>> 3 - The remnant of the patent ductus arteriosus is closed off (ligated).

> **Bottom -**
>> 4 - The two sections of the aortic arch are sutured together.
>> 5 - The ventricular septal defect is closed with a patch (shown in pink).

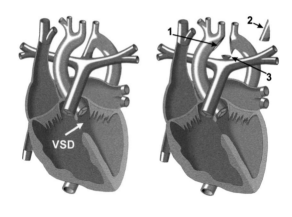

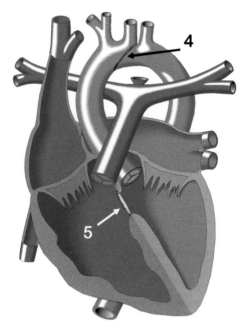

This procedure is performed to relieve complex left ventricular outflow obstruction associated with hypoplasia of the aortic valve annulus. The aortic valve is removed and an incision is made in the ventricular septum just to the patient's left of the right coronary ostium. The incised ventricular septum is patched open, which therefore widens the left ventricular outflow tract and allows replacement of the aortic valve with a larger-sized graft or prosthesis. The aortic valve is generally replaced with either a mechanical valve (Konno-Rastan), an aortic homograft, or with the patient's own pulmonic valve (Ross-Konno).

Opposite:

Figure 1 - Broken lines show the proposed sites of incisions in the aortic root. A vertical aortotomy incision will be carried down onto the infundibulum of the right ventricle (arrow 2) and into the ventricular septum (arrow 1).

Figure 2 - The aortic valve is excised at the level of the left ventricular outflow tract. Aortic "buttons" are fashioned around the coronary ostia (arrow 3), and the remainder of the proximal aortic tissue is excised. After removal of the aortic valve, the aortic annulus and left ventricular outflow tract are enlarged by incision through the annulus and down into the interventricular septum (arrow 4). This is facilitated by exposure through the right ventriculotomy incision (arrow 5).

Figure 3 - A homograft aortic valve has been sewn to the left ventricular outflow tract as a modified root replacement (arrow 6). Coronary arteries are reimplanted into the homograft root. A synthetic patch has been sewn into the ventricular incision to enlarge the subaortic left ventricular outflow tract (arrow 7).

Figure 4 - Appropriate positioning of the reimplanted coronary arteries is confirmed (arrow 8). Reconstruction is completed with a second patch, which is used to close the incision in the right ventricular infundibulum (arrow 9).

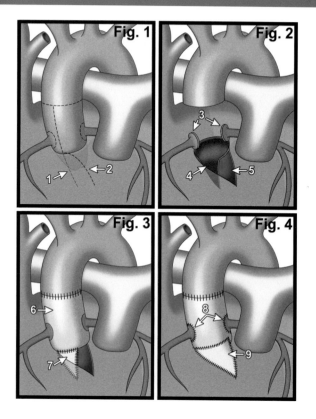

In the valve-sparing Konno procedure, the ventricular septal incision described above is made without extending it up through the aortic valve annulus. In this modification, the patient's own functional aortic valve is left in place. This procedure is appropriate for cases of complex or recurrent left ventricular outflow tract obstruction with adequate size of the aortic valve and annulus.

The coronary arteries (Fig. 4, number 8) must be re-implanted if a Konno procedure with homograft root replacement or Ross-Konno procedure is performed.

Marfan Syndrome - Aortic Root Replacement

In cases of Marfan Syndrome where the aortic root becomes enlarged to the point that the patient is at risk of dissection and rupture, the root may need to be surgically replaced. Surgery is usually indicated if the aortic root diameter approaches 5.0 cm or if the annual rate of enlargement exceeds 1.0 cm/year.

Surgical treatment of aortic root enlargement is aimed at replacing the portion of the aorta (root and proximal ascending aorta) at risk of dissection or rupture, ideally preserving the aortic valve. In cases in which the aortic valve cannot be spared, a mechanical or biological aortic prosthesis is implanted. Three of such surgical approaches are illustrated in the opposite page.

Opposite (Above): Aortic root replacement with Dacron conduit (in white). The aortic root (partially visible) and a variable portion of the ascending aorta are replaced.

Opposite (Below):

1. Valve-sparing aortic root replacement (root remodeling technique). The native valve is preserved and a scalloped graft is anastomosed to the remnants of the sinuses of Valsalva. The annulus of the non-coronary sinus is reinforced with a Teflon strip to prevent late enlargement and aortic regurgitation. The coronary arteries are (in all three techniques shown) anastomosed to the graft.

2. Valve-sparing aortic root replacement (re-implantation technique). In this technique the valve is actually reimplanted within the graft, which is anchored below the nadir of the annulus. This repair has the advantage of completely encasing the root, preventing in theory late aortic root enlargement and the development of aortic insufficiency.

3. Prosthetic valve and aortic root replacement with composite valved graft conduit

The postoperative prognosis depends on the concomitant occurrence of an aortic dissection and on whether or not the

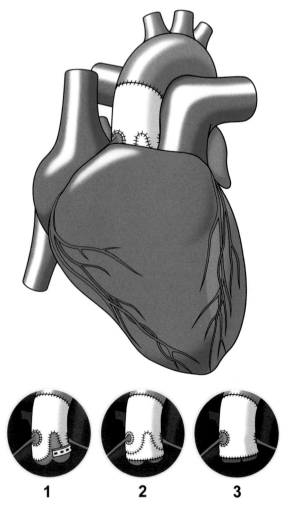

1   **2**   **3**

aortic valve was preserved or replaced. Even after surgical replacement of the aortic root, the enlargement or rupture of the remaining aorta remains a life-long risk. This, in addition to the chance of developing late aortic or mitral regurgitation, supports the need for regular clinical and imaging follow-up in patients with the Marfan syndrome.

271

If mitral valve regurgitation is minor, patients are asymptomatic and no treatment is necessary.

There are many ways to repair a more significantly regurgitant mitral valve. In some cases, mitral regurgitation may be surgically corrected by removing the area of prolapse and suturing the remaining leaflet tissue to tighten the valve opening (see illustrations).

Also, a ring (shown in white with black sutures in **Figure 6**) may be sutured into position around the valve annulus to support the repaired valve leaflets and to prevent annular dilatation. In smaller children in whom a ring cannot be used, a suture, or multiple sutures can be used to reduce the diameter of the annulus. Lastly, in cases in which valve repair is not possible, a valve replacement may be performed.

Opposite – The "Sliding Plasty" Technique:

Figure 1 - Close-up view of Mitral Valve

Figure 2 - The area of prolapse in the malformed leaflet is removed (yellow arrow indicates removal).

Figure 3 - An incision along the posterior margin of the annulus (broken line) frees the leaflet tissue so that a sliding plasty can be performed. The free edges of the remaining leaflet tissue are sutured together and then the leaflet is re-sutured to the annulus.

Figure 4 - The two portions of the posterior leaflet are sutured together; the gathered portions of the annulus adjacent to the center of the leaflet are sutured together.

Figure 5 - The posterior margin of the annulus is re-joined to the leaflet by direct suture.

Figure 6 - An annuloplasty ring (white) is sutured to the posterior periphery of the valve to support the leaflets and discourage further prolapse or annular enlargement.

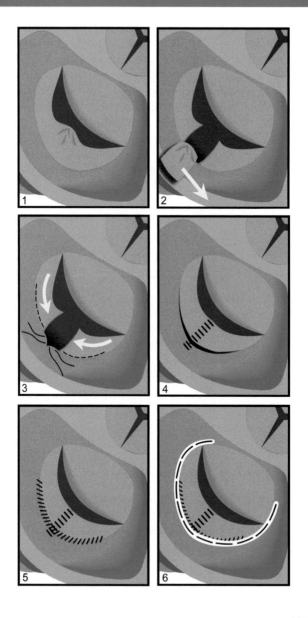

As mild cases of mitral stenosis may be asymptomatic, treatment is usually not indicated. Because of the possibility of requiring valve replacement, deferring surgical intervention as long as possible to allow implantation of a larger valve is appealing in growing children. In patients with more severe congenital mitral stenosis, medical therapy consisting of diuretics may be utilized as a bridge to definitive therapy, which is mitral valvuloplasty or replacement. In patients with rheumatic etiology of their mitral stenosis and no significant insufficiency, percutaneous balloon valvuloplasty has been utilized with success. The definitive therapy for all types of mitral stenosis that fail percutaneous[1] or open valvuloplasty is valve replacement. Post operative complications can include heart block and perivalvar leaks.

If a prosthetic mechanical valve is used, permanent anticoagulation with coumadin is necessary.

Opposite:

Top Left - Superior view of a heart with Mitral Stenosis

Top Right - Close-up view of a stenotic (undersized) mitral valve

Lower Left - The stenotic mitral valve is removed

Lower Right - A larger replacement St. Jude mitral valve is sutured into place. Compare the size of the opening of the new valve with the original, stenotic one.

---

[1]See page 190 for percutaneous mitral valvuloplasty.

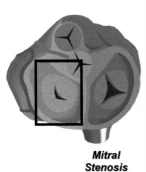

Mitral Stenosis

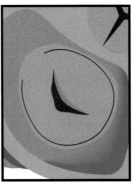

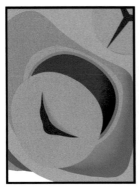

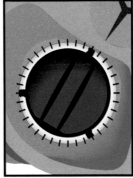

The Norwood procedure is the first step in the three stage process of reconstructive surgery for hypoplastic left heart syndrome, as well as other forms of functionally univentricular heart with systemic ventricular outflow obstruction.

The Norwood Procedure seeks to achieve three goals:

1. Amalgamation of the proximal main pulmonary artery with the aorta, and augmentation of the aortic arch in a fashion that insures unobstructed flow from the systemic ventricle to the aorta and unimpeded flow into the coronary arteries, and allows for growth of all segments of the aorta.

2. Atrial septectomy, insuring unobstructed pulmonary venous return to the systemic ventricle.

3. Regulation of pulmonary blood flow – to allow normal development and maturation of the pulmonary vasculature in anticipation of an eventual Fontan procedure.

Pulmonary blood flow may be provided and regulated by construction of a modified Blalock Taussig shunt. An alternative (commonly referred to as the Sano modification) provides pulmonary blood flow by means of interposition of a conduit (frequently polytetrafluoroethylene (PTFE)) between the systemic ventricle and pulmonary artery in place of a modified Blalock-Taussig shunt.[1]

Opposite:

Top – Norwood Procedure (blue – homograft patch, pink - expanded polytetrafluorethylene (ePTFE) shunt)

Bottom – (left) hypoplastic left heart syndrome, (right) hypoplastic left heart syndrome after the Norwood Procedure

---

[1] See page 288 for the Sano Modification of the Norwood Procedure.

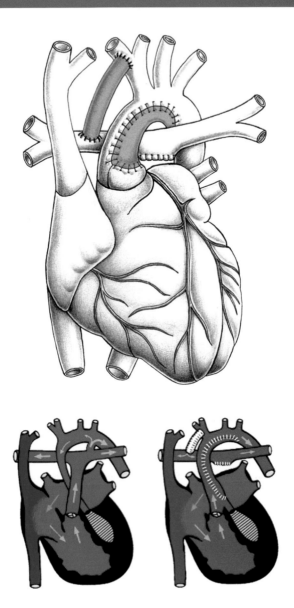

277

When a patent ductus arteriosus persists after birth, it may be ligated and, in some cases, divided. In small, premature neonates and infants, surgical interruption with titanium clips is preferred by many surgeons to ligation.

Opposite:

> **Figure 1** - External view of heart, showing the anatomical location of the patent ductus arteriosus in the other frames

> **Figure 2** - Close-up of the patent ductus arteriosus (arrow)

> **Figure 3** - Double ligation of the patent ductus arteriosus

> **Figure 4** - Division of the patent ductus arteriosus after double ligation

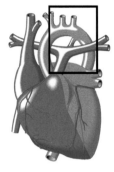

Fig. 1

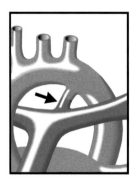

Fig. 2

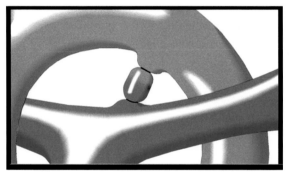

Fig. 3

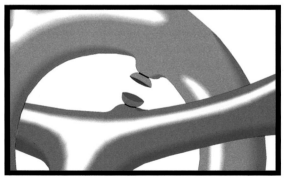

Fig. 4

279

Pulmonary Atresia: Intact Ventricular Septum

In pulmonary atresia with intact ventricular septum (PA/IVS), the critical management decision is whether or not the right ventricle is too hypoplastic to function effectively as a subpulmonary pumping chamber. Prior to palliation, pulmonary blood flow is dependent upon patency of the ductus arteriosus. When the right ventricle is diminutive and the tricuspid annulus small, this condition falls into the category of functionally univentricular heart.

In neonates with PA/IVS, if the right ventricle is too hypoplastic or if there is right ventricular dependent coronary circulation, single ventricle palliation will be necessary. This generally requires a modified Blalock-Taussig shunt[1] in the neonatal period and ultimately Fontan palliation.[2] If the tricuspid valve and right ventricle are of sufficient size, a transannular outflow patch (pink in the illustration) may sometimes be possible. This will connect the right ventricle to the main pulmonary artery. In most instances, this is combined with construction of a modified Blalock-Taussig shunt for additional pulmonary blood flow. If ventricular growth and compliance are favorable, then both the shunt and any interatrial communication can be closed at a later time, creating true biventricular circulation.

Occasionally the size of the tricuspid valve and right ventricle are sufficient to manage part, but not all of the systemic venous return. In such cases, relief of right ventricular outflow tract obstruction by means of a patch or conduit may eventually be combined with a bidirectional Glenn (superior cavopulmonary) anastomosis.[3] Thus, the right ventricle manages return from the inferior vena cava, while return from the superior vena cava is diverted directly to the lungs. Thus is commonly referred to as a "one and a half ventricle repair."

---

[1] See page 246 for the Modified Blalock-Taussig shunt.
[2] See pages 258-261 for the Fontan Procedure.
[3] See page 262 for the Glenn Shunt Procedure.

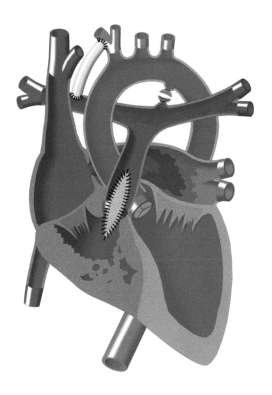

Above:

Patch angioplasty of an atretic pulmonary artery
through the insertion of a patch (shown in pink) and a
modified Blalock-Taussig Shunt (shown in light blue).
Note ligation of patent ductus arteriosus (PDA).

In some patients (small patients, multiple co-morbidities, multiple co-morbidities, anomalous coronaries etc.), complete intracardiac repair may best be deferred or may not feasible (functionally univentricular heart). To reduce pulmonary blood flow, a constricting band (Damman-Muller procedure) is placed around the main pulmonary artery above the valve. This reduces the artery diameter (and blood flow) and achieves a more balanced pulmonary blood flow to systemic blood flow ratio, minimizing pulmonary overcirculation and avoiding the development of pulmonary hypertension. The band serves its purpose until somatic growth has exceeded the critical diameter of the band and the child becomes increasingly cyanotic. At reoperation or second-stage palliation, the band is removed and the pulmonary artery reconstructed.

Opposite - Top:

Pulmonary band treatment of ventricular septal defect

Opposite - Bottom:

Left - Coarctation of the aorta with a large apical muscular ventricular septal defect

Right - After coarctation repair and insertion of a pulmonary band (indicated by white arrow) with the ventricular septal defect left open.

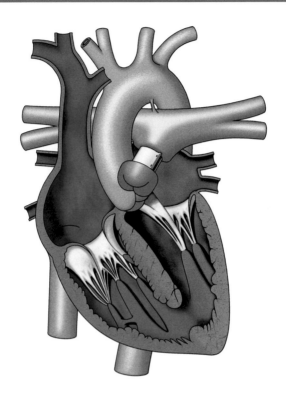

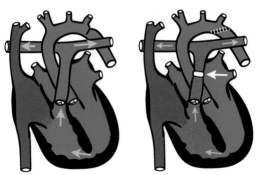

283

In patients with pulmonary stenosis not amenable to trans-catheter intervention, the surgical approach depends on the location of the stenosis. If the stenosis is supravalvular, the pulmonary artery can be widened with a "hood" of pericardium or prosthetic material.

If the stenosis is subvalvular, the obstructing muscle can be excised through the tricuspid valve or directly through an incision into the right ventricular ouflow tract. The latter can then be augmented with a patch as mentioned above to further expand the outflow tract diameter.

Should the stenosis involve the valve with a small annulus of the pulmonary valve, the incision is carried out proximal and distal to the valve, and the right ventricular outflow tract is augmented with a transannular patch (light blue in bottom diagram **opposite**).

Opposite:

>   **Top** - Repair of a stenotic pulmonary artery through the insertion of a patch on the main pulmonary artery

>   **Bottom** - Repair of a stenotic pulmonary artery through the insertion of a transannular patch (shown in light blue). The lower part of the patch is sutured to the outer wall of the right ventricle.

Below: Internal view of supravalvular pulmonary stenosis

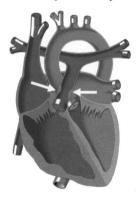

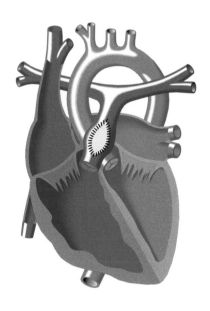

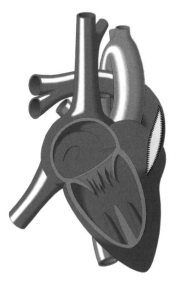

In some cases where an aortic valve replacement is required, it is possible to use the patient's own pulmonary valve and move it into the aortic position. The patient's right ventricular outflow tract (where the pulmonary artery root has been procured) is reconstructed with a pulmonary homograft. As part of the procedure, the coronary arteries need to be detached and re-implanted on the autograft.

In cases where the aortic valve is undersized, thickened, or malformed (valvular aortic stenosis), an initial palliative treatment involves the widening of the opening to allow a greater flow of blood into the aorta. This may be achieved either by surgery (open valvotomy) or a transcatheter balloon valvuloplasty.[1] This initial approach allows the postponement of a more extensive operation such as the Ross procedure or other type of aortic valve replacement. At the time of valve replacement, mechanical or bioprosthetic replacement valves (xenografts and homografts) are alternatives to the pulmonary autograft (Ross procedure). Homografts are most commonly used in cases of aortic root abscess and severe endocarditis.

In the Ross Procedure, the patient's own pulmonary valve root is transposed into the aortic position, the coronary arteries are reimplanted into the autograft and a pulmonary homograft is used to replace the harvested pulmonary root.

The Ross procedure is the only aortic valve replacement option that provides the possibility of growth and thus is particularly appealing in infants and children. The procedure should not be considered in patients with aortic root enlargement secondary to connective tissue disorders, and should be selectively utilized in patients with bicuspid aortic valve and with aortic insufficiency as the primary pathology.

---

[1] See page 188 for aortic valvuloplasty.

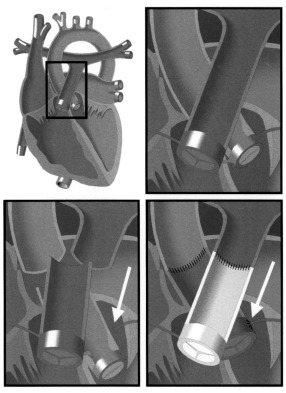

Upper Left - Overall view of heart, Insert: aortic and pulmonary roots.

Upper Right - Close-up of the stenotic aorta behind the pulmonary artery

Lower Left - Narrowed section of aorta is removed and the coronary arteries separated from it (arrow); the proximal portion of the pulmonary artery, including the pulmonary valve, is removed.

Lower Right - The pulmonary valve and lower portion of the pulmonary artery are sutured to the aorta. A homograft (light blue) is sutured to the pulmonary artery. The coronary arteries are sutured to the neoaorta (arrow).

The Sano modification includes all of the features of the Norwood procedure (see **page 276**), but it incorporates the use of a right ventricle to pulmonary artery conduit as an alternative to the Blalock-Taussig shunt commonly used in the Norwood procedure. This prevents diastolic runoff of systemic blood into the pulmonary arteries providing a higher diastolic blood pressure and, presumably, better coronary perfusion.

Most often, the conduit used in the Sano modification of the Norwood procedure is a simple non-valved tube graft of polytetrafluoroethylene (PTFE). Some surgeons prefer to incorporate a very small homograft or allograft valve, to reduce conduit insufficiency and limit systemic ventricular volume load.

Opposite: Sano modification of Norwood Procedure

pink - homograft
blue - right ventricle to pulmonary artery conduit

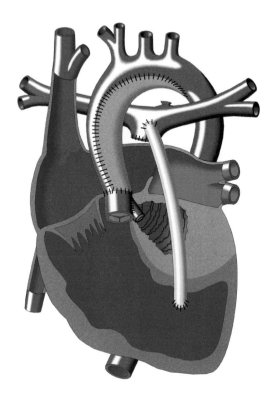

289

Septal Myectomy

There are various treatments for hypertrophic obstructive cardiomyopathy. These include medical therapy with beta blockers and calcium channel blockers, which slow the heart rate and increase the diastolic filling time of the ventricle, thereby decreasing the left ventricular outflow tract obstruction. Most patients benefit in terms of symptoms from oral medications.

For those patients with significant symptoms or severe left ventricular outflow tract obstruction, surgical reduction (septal myectomy) of the ventricular septum is indicated. More recently, in selected adult patients with hypertrophic cardiomyopathy, percutaneous alcohol septal ablation has been demonstrated to be of benefit in gradient reduction.

Dual chamber pacing may provide a modest benefit in symptom relief in these patients. However, Implantable Cardiac Defibrillators (ICD) have been advocated for use in patients at high risk for sudden death.

During the septal myectomy operation, the atrio-ventricular conduction system is particularly vulnerable to iatrogenic injury due to its proximity to the area of myectomy. Therefore complete heart block is a potential complication of this procedure.

Opposite - Top:

Internal view of a heart with hypertrophic cardiomyopathy. Note the narrowing of the outflow tract from the left ventricle into the aorta (arrow).

Opposite - Bottom:

The outflow tract is widened by the removal of excess ventricular septal tissue (arrow).

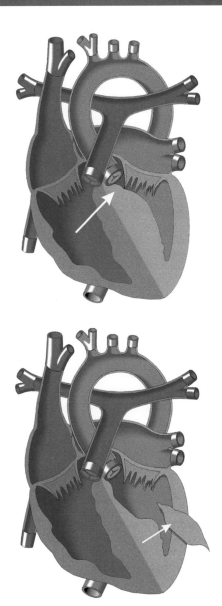

There are various ways in which an anomalous left coronary artery arising from the pulmonary artery may be surgically treated. Most often, the left coronary artery is simply detached from the pulmonary artery and sutured directly onto the aorta.[1]

An alternative is the Takeuchi Procedure. In the Takeuchi Procedure (see illustrations), a small aorto-pulmonary window is created and a baffle is placed within the pulmonary artery tunneling blood from the aorta to the anomalous orifice of the left coronary artery within the pulmonary artery.

To create this baffle, or tunnel, Takeuchi used a flap fashioned from the anterior wall of the main pulmonary artery. In a simplified modification of the procedure, the tunnel is fashioned from autologous pericardium or prosthetic material such as polytetrafluoroethylene (ePTFE). The main pulmonary artery is generally enlarged with a patch.

This procedure is potentially useful when the ostium of the anomalous coronary artery arises in a very lateral or distant location from the aortic root, making transfer of the coronary to the aortic root difficult.

Opposite:

> **Top** – Internal view of anomalous left coronary artery from the pulmonary artery. Rectangle shows area of close-up views.

> **Lower Left** – An aorto-pulmonary window (indicated by arrow) is created in the wall of the pulmonary artery.

> **Lower Right** – A conduit (light blue) is sutured on the posterior interior wall of the pulmonary artery to carry blood from the aorta into the left coronary artery. Arrow shows direction of blood flow from aorta through conduit.

---

[1] See Reimplantation Repair, page 228.

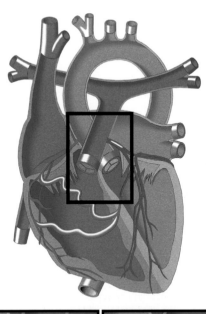

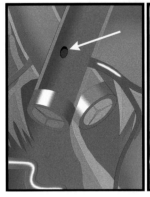
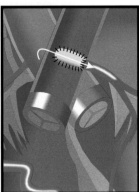

293

Tetralogy of Fallot involves four morphologic findings:

1. A large malalignment ventricular septal defect

2. An enlarged aorta which overrides the ventricular septum

3. An obstructed right ventricular outflow tract, caused by infundibular and/or valvar pulmonary stenosis

4. Hypertrophy of the right ventricle

In fact, all four of these elements of tetralogy of Fallot are manifestations or consequences of the single unifying feature of the anomaly - hypoplasia of the infundibulum of the right ventricle which is associated with anterosuperior deviation of the conal septum.

The objectives of reparative surgery for tetralogy of Fallot are closure of the ventricular septal defect and relief of right ventricular outflow obstruction. This latter goal is accomplished by resection of obstructing infundibular muscle bands and right ventricular outflow patch reconstruction as necessary. The patch may or may not require extension across the annulus of the pulmonary valve (transannular patch).

Complete repair (described above) may sometimes be deferred in the symptomatic neonate because of patient size, small pulmonary arteries or other defects. In this circumstance, initial palliation is with a modified Blalock-Taussig shunt with subsequent complete repair which usually is accomplished at 4 to 12 months of age.

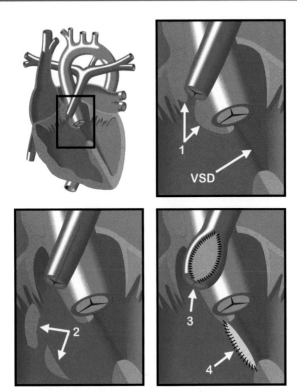

Above: Tetralogy of Fallot Surgery

Top Left: Internal view of a heart with tetralogy of Fallot, showing position of other frames

Top Right: Close-up view showing infundibular stenosis (**1**) and ventricular septal defect (VSD)

Lower Left: Obstructing muscle tissue (**2**) is surgically removed. The red line shows the incision of the stenotic pulmonary artery for widening and patching.

Lower Right: (**3**) - Widened and patched pulmonary artery; (**4**) - patched ventricular septal defect (patch shown in pink).

Truncus arteriosus is generally repaired during the first weeks of life. Surgical treatment of this defect involves the separation of the pulmonary arteries from the truncus arteriosus. The pulmonary arteries are then connected to the right ventricle – most often with a valved conduit (light blue in the illustration), usually a pulmonary or aortic homograft (cryopreserved human tissue) or bovine jugular vein valved conduit. Porcine valved Dacron conduits may also be used.

The ventricular septal defect is closed with a patch, and the point of the detachment of the pulmonary arteries from the common arterial trunk is closed directly or with a patch.

The truncus now assumes the functional role of the aorta, carrying blood from the left ventricle to the body. The truncal valve may be stenotic/insufficient, with repair or replacement at this time or later in cases of late regurgitation.

In a subset of patients, the common arterial trunk is associated with interruption or obstruction of the aortic arch. Though a high risk procedure, definitive repair including arch reconstruction and repair of common arterial trunk is the preferred approach.

Opposite:

> **Top Left** - Internal view of a heart with truncus arteriosus (TA). Note also the ventricular septal defect (VSD).

Top Right:
> **1** - The connection between the pulmonary artery and the truncus arteriosus is divided by the removal of a section of the pulmonary artery.
>
> **2** - The resulting defect in the truncus is closed with sutures.

Bottom -
> **1** - A valved tube, or conduit (light blue) connects the pulmonary artery branches to the right ventricle.
>
> **2** - The ventricular septal defect is patched (shown in pink).

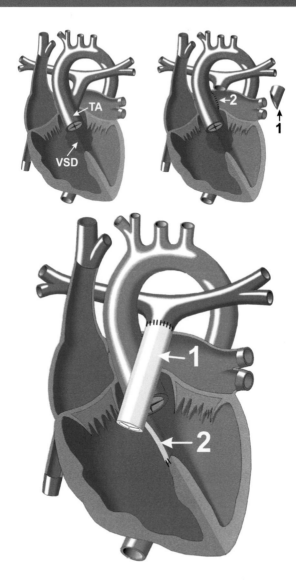

Vascular Ring Repair - Double Aortic Arch

Almost all vascular rings are approached through a left thoracotomy.

Surgical treatment of the most common forms of this defect (e. g. double aortic arch) involves the ligation and division of one of the components of the double aortic arch. This procedure breaks the constricting ring around the trachea and esophagus.

Sometimes, one of the branches is atretic, with no blood flowing through it. In this case, it is simply ligated and divided.

In cases where blood flows through both branches, the smaller vessel is ligated and divided at a point between the subclavian artery (SA in top illustration) and where the smaller branch joins the larger branch to form the descending aorta.

Opposite:

   Top - Internal view of a heart with double aortic arch. (SA – subclavian artery)

   Middle - Double ligation of smaller branch of the aorta (shown by arrow)

   Bottom - Division of smaller branch of the aorta (shown by arrow)

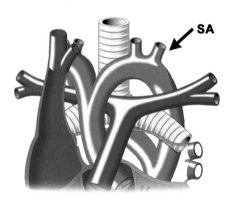

SA

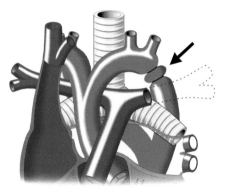

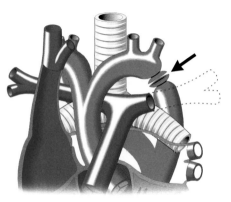

Treatment of a vascular ring with right aortic arch (RAA) and left-sided patent ductus arteriosus (PDA) involves the division of the ligamentum arteriosum. In addition, Kommerell's diverticulum is usually removed from the left subclavian artery, which is then closed with sutures. Alternatively, it can be tacked to the pre-vertebral fascia (diverticulopexy), avoiding compression to trachea or esophagus. These procedures break the constricting ring around the trachea and esophagus.

Opposite:

Top Left - External view of a heart with vascular ring.

Top Right - Close-up view of vascular ring showing the subclavian artery (SA), ligamentum arteriosum (LA), and Kommerell's diverticulum (KD).

Lower Left - The vascular ring is broken by the removal of the Kommerell's diverticulum.

Lower Right - The pulmonary artery and subclavian artery are closed with sutures.

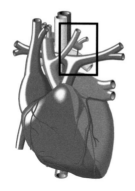

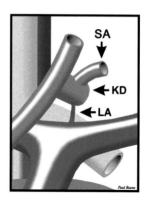

SA

KD

LA

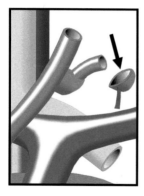

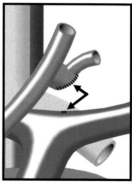

Closure of ventricular septal defect(s) is the most commonly performed open heart operation for congenital heart disease.

Ventricular septal defects are generally closed with a patch. According to the location of the defect, VSDs can be approached either through the right atrium, the right ventricle, or through the pulmonary valve. Very occasionally, a VSD is approached through the aortic valve. Larger holes may be closed with patches made of pericardium or of synthetic materials such as Dacron or expanded polytetrafluoroethylene (ePTFE).

Knowledge of the disposition of the specialized conduction tissue relative to the margins of a ventricular septal defect is critical, in order to avoid the completion of surgically induced complete heart block.

Opposite:

Top - Internal view from the right side of a heart with a ventricular septal defect (VSD)

Bottom - A patch (shown in pink) made of pericardium or a synthetic material is used to cover the VSD.

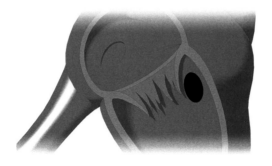

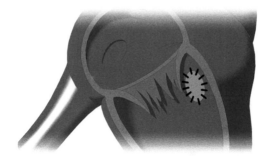

Some shunt procedures that were performed in the past:

Opposite:

> **Top left:** Tetralogy of Fallot with classic Blalock-Taussig Shunt. The subclavian artery is divided distally and attached directly to the right pulmonary artery.

> **Top right:** Tetralogy of Fallot with Waterston Shunt. A fenestration type connection from the ascending aorta to right pulmonary artery.

> **Bottom left:** Apical left ventricle to descending aorta conduit.

> **Bottom right:** Tetralogy of Fallot with a central shunt. An ascending aorta to main pulmonary artery anastomosis using a small prosthetic tube graft.

Below:

> **Left:** Tricuspid atresia with Potts shunt. A fenestration type connection from the descending aorta to left pulmonary artery.

> **Right:** Tricuspid atresia with classical (unidirectional) Glenn Shunt. A superior vena cava to isolated right pulmonary artery anastomosis.

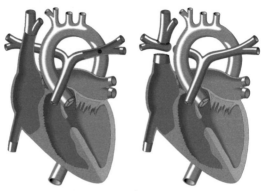

Potts Shunt   **Glenn Shunt**

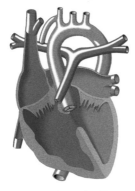

Blalock-Taussig Shunt

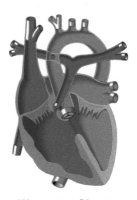

Waterston Shunt

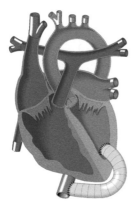

Apical LV - Aortic Conduit

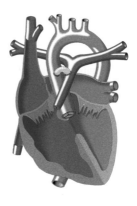

Central Shunt

CHAPTER 8. **CARDIAC ICU TOPICS**

By Stacie B. Peddy, MD, David S. Cooper. MD, MPH,
Jeffrey P. Jacobs, MD, and Marshall L. Jacobs, MD

INTRAOPERATIVE EVENTS

Cardiopulmonary Bypass (CPB) – Cardiopulmonary bypass is defined as the process of diverting venous blood from a patient's heart and lungs to a gas exchange system for the addition of oxygen, removal of carbon dioxide, and subsequent re-infusion to the patient's arterial system.

Cardiopulmonary bypass uses the heart and lung bypass machine. The expression "open heart surgery" is commonly used in reference to surgery that is performed with cardiopulmonary bypass (CPB) support. Operations performed without CPB are generally referred to as "closed heart operations." While these terms are not precise or literal in their descriptions, they have nonetheless found their way into common usage.

Cardiopulmonary bypass support is accomplished using a circuit consisting of a pump, an oxygenator, a heat exchanger, and a reservoir (see **Figure 1, page 311**). Venous blood is drained from the heart by a cannula in the right atrium or separate cannulas in the superior and inferior venae cavae. Venous blood drains into a reservoir and then passes through the pump (either a roller head pump or a centrifugal pump), through an oxygenator, where oxygen and carbon dioxide are titrated, and then through a heat exchanger (the order in which blood passes through these essential elements of the circuit can vary with the design of the system). The blood then returns to the patient via an arterial cannula which is most often placed in the ascending aorta, but may be placed in another systemic artery such as a femoral artery. The bypass circuit is primed with fluid, consisting of a physiologic electrolyte solution (crystalloid) alone or in combination with packed red blood cells or whole blood.

It is a common practice to cool the blood circulating through the bypass circuit to achieve a patient temperature of 28 to 32 degrees centigrade (moderate hypothermia), or even cooler. Lower temperatures enable the patient to tolerate rates of flow that are less than the normal cardiac output. After the cardiac repair is completed, the circulating blood, and thus the patient, is rewarmed to achieve normothermia.

> *Cardiopulmonary Bypass Time* - The total number of minutes that systemic return is diverted into the cardiopulmonary bypass (CPB) circuit and returned to the systemic system. (Ref. 3, p. 337)

Aortic Cross Clamp – Intracardiac repairs are generally performed using the technique of aortic cross-clamping and cardioplegic arrest. After systemic cooling has been achieved, a clamp is applied to occlude the ascending aorta, proximal to the aortic cannula. A cardioplegic solution is then injected into the aortic root and thus the coronary circulation, to arrest and protect the heart.

> *Aortic Cross Clamp Time* - The total number of minutes that the coronary circulation is mechanically isolated from systemic circulation, either by an aortic cross clamp or systemic circulatory arrest. This time period (Cross Clamp Time) includes all intervals of intermittent or continuous cardioplegia administration. (Ref. 3, p. 337)

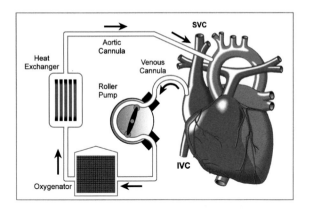

Figure 1: Cardiopulmonary Bypass (CPB)

IVC - inferior vena cava, SVC - superior vena cava

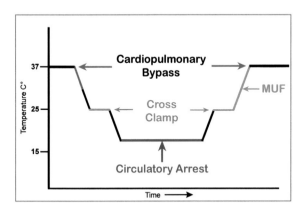

**Figure 2: Patient Temperature During
Intra-Operative Events**

MUF - Modified ultrafiltration

311

Circulatory Arrest – The technique of deep hypothermia with circulatory arrest (DHCA) is used in some operations, particularly those that involve reconstruction of the aortic arch, or more generally in very small infants. After cooling the patient on cardiopulmonary bypass to a core temperature of 16 to 20 degrees centigrade, the entire circulation is arrested (CPB turned off), which facilitates aortic arch repair or intracardiac repair in a completely bloodless field. Deep hypothermia provides protection during this period of total body ischemia. Once the surgical repair is completed, cardiopulmonary bypass flow is resumed and the patient is rewarmed (**Figure 2**, page 311).

> *Circulatory Arrest Time* - The total number of minutes of complete cessation of blood flow to the patient. This time period (Circulatory Arrest Time) excludes any periods of cerebral perfusion. (Ref. 3, p. 337)

Regional Cerebral Perfusion – This technique involves continuous perfusion of the brain while the remainder of the body is subjected to a period of hypothermic circulatory arrest. In pediatric cardiac surgery, antegrade regional perfusion is used more commonly than retrograde cerebral perfusion. Antegrade regional cerebral perfusion is generally accomplished either by direct placement of the arterial cannula in the innominate or right common carotid artery, or by inserting the cannula into a small PTFE graft that has been sewn to one of these vessels. Retrograde cerebral perfusion is generally accomplished with the placement of a perfusion cannula in the superior vena cava. Used in operations that include aortic arch reconstruction, regional cerebral perfusion has intuitive appeal, but has not been shown to be superior to DHCA.

Ultrafiltration – Hemofiltration can be carried out throughout the period of cardiopulmonary bypass (conventional ultra-filtration) or immediately after termination of bypass support (modified ultrafiltration or MUF).

Modified ultrafiltration is a technique designed to hemoconcentrate the patient and the cardiopulmonary bypass circuit after the cessation of cardiopulmonary bypass.

MUF is a way to decrease total body water, raise the hematocrit, and remove inflammatory mediators. In some studies, use of MUF has been shown to improve postoperative hemodynamics, decrease postoperative blood loss, and contribute to fewer days of intubation in the ICU.

Transesophageal Echocardiogram (TEE) – TEE is echocardiography with the transducer in the esophagus. TEE is used in most open heart cases to assess the heart before and after repair. At the completion of surgery, it allows assessment of ventricular function and of the status of the repair. Miniaturized probes facilitate the performance of TEE in infants weighing 3 kg or more, and in some instances in infants weighing less than 3 kg.

ASSESSMENT OF THE POST-OPERATIVE PATIENT

Understand the pre-operative anatomy and physiology.

- What was the detailed preoperative cardiac diagnosis? In what ways were the anatomy and physiology different from normal?
- Cyanosis? Pulmonary over-circulation? Congestive Heart Failure (CHF)?
- Effects of the cardiac anatomy and physiology on the other organ systems?
- Pre-operative medications - indications, side effects?
- Why was this patient operated on now?

The Surgery

- What were the operative findings?
- What anesthetic technique was used?
- What is the nature of the surgical repair?

Outcome of Surgery

- Were all of the objectives of the operation achieved?
- How are the anatomy and physiology different now relative to pre-op status?
- Are there any new or residual hemodynamic problems: cardiac conduction and rhythm disorders, residual defects (intracardiac shunts, outflow tract obstruction, valvar stenosis or regurgitation), diminished myocardial function?
- What pharmacologic support, if any, has been used since separation from cardiopulmonary bypass?
- Has sternal wound closure been completed or deferred?

The Conduction System

- Compare pre-operative and post-operative 12 lead ECG.
- How was the conduction system affected by the surgical procedure?
- Is this patient at risk for JET (Junctional Ectopic Tachycardia) by age and/or cardiac lesion?
- Were there any arrhythmias coming off CPB or in the operating room? What was the treatment?
- What temporary or permanent pacing wires (leads) were placed during surgery, and how are they being used?

Pulmonary Function

- How was pulmonary function affected by anesthesia and surgery?
- What mode of mechanical ventilation to utilize?
- What is the expected range of systemic arterial saturation (sPO_2)?
- Planned early extubation or continued ventilatory support?

Other Organ Systems

- How were these organs affected by the anesthesia, surgery and cardiopulmonary bypass?
- Renal: adequate urine output, hematuria, hemoglobinuria?
- Hematologic: bleeding, measurable coagulation parameters, optimal hematocrit?
- Integument: intact and adequately perfused on all body parts, sufficient padding to avoid pressure injury?
- Central nervous system: anesthesia, muscle relaxation, emergence from anesthesia, seizures or other evidence of neurologic abnormality?

INTRACARDIAC MONITORING LINES & OTHER "ACCESSORIES" OF THE POST OPERATIVE PATIENT

Chest X-Ray - Taken upon admission to the ICU, to evaluate ETT placement, and other hardware including central lines, chest tubes, mediastinal tubes, temporary pacing wires, etc.

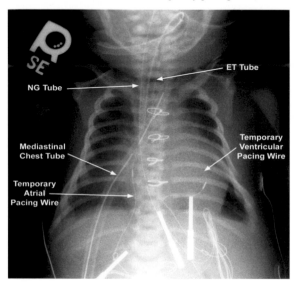

Figure 3 - Chest X-Ray

Central Venous Lines - Central lines are usually placed in the internal jugular, subclavian or femoral veins after the induction of anesthesia. In neonates they are often placed in the umbilical vein. Used for administration of vasoactive infusions, fluids, parenteral nutrition, and measurement of central venous pressures. If the tip ends at the junction of the Superior Vena Cava and the Right Atrium, it can be used to sample a mixed venous saturation. There is a risk of causing atrial arrhythmias if the tip is in the right atrium.

Intracardiac Lines

- Right atrial (RA), left atrial (LA) and pulmonary artery (PA) catheters

- LA line - usually inserted via the right upper pulmonary vein or LA appendage
  - Helpful to assess systemic ventricular or atrioventricular (AV) valve function (often used with extensive mitral valve repair)

- PA line - Inserted in right ventricular (RV) outflow tract and fed across pulmonary valve (PV), or inserted directly into PA.
  - Can sample a Mixed Venous Oxygen Saturation
  - Can evaluate PA pressure & Pulmonary Vascular Resistance (PVR). Measurement of PVR is useful in patients with pre-op pulmonary hypertension.
  - Upon removal, a PA pullback can be done to assess residual Right Ventricular Outflow Tract (RVOT) obstruction, if the line is placed via the RVOT.

Chest Tube and Mediastinal Drains

- There should be concern for surgical bleeding if output greater than 5-10 cc/kg/hr, but a sudden decrease in output is also a concern for clot formation and the development of pericardial or pleural effusions.

- Pleural drainage that is creamy or cloudy, especially if the change is temporally related to initiation of feeds, is likely a chylous effusion (chylothorax) from damage to the thoracic duct. Thoracic duct injury is more common during surgeries involving arch reconstruction or manipulation.

  Chylothorax - Presence of lymphatic fluid in the pleural space, commonly secondary to leakage from the thoracic duct or one of its main tributaries. Thoracocentesis is the gold standard for diagnosis and generally reveals a predominance of lymphocytes and/or a triglyceride level greater than 110 mg/dL.(Ref. 3, p. 337)

317

Clinical Correlates - Table 1

Clinical Condition	RA/CVP	LA	BP
Tamponade	↑	↑	↓
Low CO (with euvolemia)	↑	↑	↓
Hypovolemia	↓	↓	↔ ↓
AV Block	↑	↑	↓

RA/CVP - Right Atrial/Central Venous Pressure
LA - Left Atrium, BP - Blood Pressure
CO - Cardiac Output, AV - Atrioventricular

LOW CARDIAC OUTPUT SYNDROME (LCOS)

LCOS is one of the most important predictors of poor outcome after surgery for CHD.[1] Neonates and infants undergoing biventricular repair of CHD with cardiopulmonary bypass (CPB) have a predictable drop in cardiac index, 32% below baseline at 9-12 hrs after cross-clamp removal, with a commensurate increase in systemic vascular resistance (SVR) and pulmonary vascular resistance (PVR).[2] Longer duration of CPB and younger age are risk factors for low cardiac output syndrome.[3]

LCOS is diagnosed by a combination of clinical and laboratory data.

Signs of Low Cardiac Output Syndrome (LCOS)
- tachycardia
- oliguria
- delayed/poor capillary refill
- hypotension
- low mixed venous O_2 saturation (30% less than the arterial O_2 saturation)
- metabolic or lactic acidosis
- A mixed venous O_2 saturation that is 20-25% less than the arterial O_2 saturation indicates adequate CO and oxygen delivery

Treatment of LCOS (with normal volume status)
- Inotropic Support - calcium (esp. in neonates), dopamine, dobutamine, epinephrine, milrinone
- Chronotropic Support - isoproterenol or temporary pacing
- Afterload Reduction - nitroprusside, milrinone
- Mechanical Circulatory Support

---

[1] Parr et al, *Circulation,* 1975

[2] Wernovsky et al., *Circulation,* 1995

[3] Tweddell et al, *Ann Thorac Surg,* 2000

PULMONARY HYPERTENSION AND PULMONARY VASCULAR RESISTANCE (PVR)

Pulmonary Hypertension is defined as mean pulmonary artery pressure of greater than 25 mm Hg after the first few weeks of life. Of note, pulmonary hypertension is not the same as increased PVR.

PVR is defined as resistance to blood flow within the lungs, which is influenced by the anatomy of the vascular bed, vascular tone, pulmonary blood flow (Qp) and left atrial pressure.

• PVR = (PA pressure - LA pressure)/Qp

Postoperative pulmonary hypertension - Clinically significant elevation of pulmonary arterial pressure, requiring intervention such as nitric oxide, or other therapies. Typically, the mean pulmonary arterial pressure is greater than 25mmHg in the presence of a normal pulmonary arterial occlusion pressure (wedge pressure). (Ref. 3, p. 337)

Postoperative pulmonary hypertensive crisis (PA pressure > systemic pressure) - An acute state of inadequate systemic perfusion associated with pulmonary hypertension, when the pulmonary arterial pressure is greater than the systemic arterial pressure. (Ref. 3, p. 337)

How to identify those at risk for Post-operative Pulmonary Hypertension
• Patients with increased PVR pre-operatively
• Infants in the first several days of life
• Patients with pulmonary venous hypertension (e. g. Total Anomalous Pulmonary Venous Return)
• Older children with uncorrected CHD leading to increased PVR
• Patients with systemic PA pressure

Conditions that Increase or Decrease PVR
- ↑ **PVR** - Hypoxia, hypercarbia/acidosis, polycythemia, atelectasis, hyperinflation, CPB, agitation
- ↓ **PVR** - Oxygen, alkalosis, normal functional residual capacity (FRC), low hematocrit, nitric oxide

Treatment/Prevention of Pulmonary Hypertension
- Analgesia and sedation
- Oxygen
- Appropriate amount of PEEP to maintain FRC (functional residual capacity)
- Serum alkalinization
- Inhaled nitric oxide
- Avoidance of unnecessary endotracheal tube (ETT) suctioning

CARDIOPULMONARY INTERACTIONS

Effect of positive pressure ventilation on Right Atrium (RA) and Right Ventricle (RV)

- Increased intrathoracic pressure → increase in RA pressure → decreased venous return to RA → decreased RV preload → decreased RV output
- Lung volumes above or below FRC → increased PVR → increased RV afterload that can lead to decreased RV function

Effect of positive pressure ventilation on Left Atrium (LA) and Left Ventricle (LV)

- Increased intrathoracic pressure → decrease in LV transmural pressure → decreased LV afterload → increased LV output

Effect of positive pressure ventilation on Single Ventricle Physiology

- Increased intrathoracic pressure → increased common atrial pressure → increased transpulmonary gradient → decreased passive PBF in post-operative cavopulmonary anastomosis/Glenn or Hemi-Fontan or Fontan patients
- Lung volumes above or below FRC → increased PVR → decreased shunt flow in post-operative Stage I Norwood patients
- Lung volumes above or below FRC → increased PVR → decreased passive PBF in post-operative cavopulmonary anastomosis/Glenn or Hemi-Fontan patients

RENAL REPLACEMENT THERAPIES IN THE CICU

Indications: hypervolemia, hyperkalemia, metabolic acidosis, azotemia, neurological complications, calcium/phosphorus imbalance

Indications	PD	HD	CAVH	CVVH
Fluid Removal	+	++	++	++
Urea and Cr Clearance	+	++	+	++
K Clearance	++	++	+	++
Complications	PD	HD	CAVH	CVVH
Bleeding/ Heparinization	-	+	+	+
Peritonitis	+	-	-	-
Protein Loss	++	-	-	-
Hypotension	+	++	+	+
Respiratory Compromise	+	possible	-	-

Table 2 - Comparisons of Renal Replacement Modalities
Peritoneal Dialysis (PD), Hemodialysis (HD), Continuous Arteriovenous Hemofiltration (CAVH), Continuous Venovenous Hemofiltration (CVVH), Creatinine (Cr), Potassium (K)

(Modified from Fivush BA, Neu AM, Parekh R, Maxwell LG, Racusen LC, White JRM and Nichols DG: Renal Function and Heart Disease. In Nichols DG (ed): Critical Heart Disease in Infants and Children, 2nd ed. Philadelphia: Mosby Elsevier, 2006, p 121.)

Peritoneal Dialysis

• Ultrafiltration (UF) - removal of volume
  – Determined by solute concentration gradient, blood supply, dialysate composition, and distribution

• Solute Clearance - removal of urea, Cr, and K
  – Determined by osmotic gradients

323

To Improve Ultrafiltration	To Improve Solute Clearance
↑ Glucose Concentration	↑ dialysate volume
↑ frequency of cycles	↑ K and Urea - frequency of cycles
↑ dialysate volume	↓ Phosphorus - frequency of cycles

Table 3 - Peritoneal Dialysis

Hemodialysis

- UF & Diffusion - occurs across a man-made semipermeable membrane between blood and dialysate

- Primary determinant of UF - Hydrostatic pressure across membrane

- Diffusion of substance from blood to dialysate determined by: solute concentration, dialyzer (surface area and permeability) and flow rates

CAVH/CVVH

- Requires venous +/- arterial access

- Provides UF and some solute removal (to increase solute removal must provide dialysis – CAVHD/CVVHD - by providing filtration replacement fluid or add adding counter current dialysis)

Opposite: Figure 4 - "A-Wire Tracing" The LA, LL, and RL leads are attached to the body while the RA lead is attached to the atrial wire. This configuration enhances atrial activity in all leads except lead III.

POST-OPERATIVE PACEMAKER AND CARDIAC ARRHYTHMIAS

Temporary Pacemaker

- Atrial wires usually on the patient's right side (always confirm)

- Ventricular wires usually on the patient's left side (always confirm)

- Can be used as a diagnostic tool to assess the relationship (ratio) between the atrial and ventricular electrical activity by creating an "A wire tracing" (see **Figure 4, below**)

- Can be used as a therapeutic tool for bradycardia, heart block, or tachyarrhythmias (overdrive-pacing)

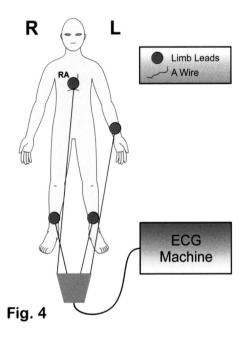

Fig. 4

POST-OPERATIVE PACEMAKER AND CARDIAC ARRHYTHMIAS (continued)

Junctional Ectopic Tachycardia (JET)

A potentially lethal automatic tachyarrhythmia, JET has an increased incidence following repair of tetralogy of Fallot, atrioventricular septal defect (AV canal), ventricular septal defect (VSD), d-transposition of the great arteries (d-TGA), and total anomalous pulmonary venous return (TAPVR). Younger age (<2 years of age) and longer CPB and aortic cross clamp time are also risk factors for JET. JET is associated with prolonged ventilator time and CICU length of stay.

- **Diagnosis** - Commonly, there is atrioventricular (AV) dissociation with more QRS complexes than P waves on ECG, rates of > 180, and narrow QRS morphology. Occasionally, there is AV association with retrograde P waves on ECG. Additionally, cannon A-waves can be seen on the CVP tracing (ADD CVP trace). JET adversely affects blood pressure because of the rapid rate and lack of AV synchrony.

- **Treatment** - Treatment should be initiated as early as possible because it is associated with faster time to control of rate and rhythm, less amiodarone, and shorter CICU length of stay. Treatment consists of sedation, core cooling, decrease or discontinuation of catecholamine agents, correction of electrolytes (K^+, Ca^{+2}, Mg^{+2}), overdrive atrial pacing (rate > junctional rate) to restore AV synchrony, and/or IV Amiodarone.

Opposite:

Figure 5 - Junctional ectopic tachycardia in a post-operative patient. Arrows (see top tracing) demonstrate non-conducted P waves buried in the T wave and **arrow heads** indicate a lack of P waves before the QRS, demonstrating AV dissociation.

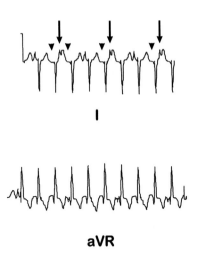

I

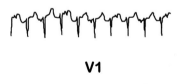

aVR

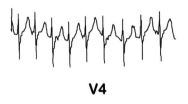

V1

V4

Fig. 5

327

MECHANICAL CIRCULATORY SUPPORT

Indications:

1) severe acute reversible cardiac dysfunction (myo-carditis, etc.)
2) severe acute reversible pulmonary dysfunction
3) cardiac arrest
4) intractable arrhythmia
5) unresponsive pulmonary hypertension
6) bridge to transplantation
7) inability to wean from cardiopulmonary bypass after heart surgery
8) hemodynamic instability after heart surgery requiring escalating inotropic support

Types of mechanical circulatory support:

1) extracorporeal membrane oxygenation (ECMO)
2) ventricular assist devices – RVAD, LVAD, BiVAD extracorporeal, paracorporeal, intracorporeal (adults only)
3) intra-aortic balloon counterpulsation

Extracorporeal membrane oxygenation is defined as the process of diverting venous blood from a patient to a gas exchange system for the addition of oxygen, removal of carbon dioxide, and subsequent re-infusion to the patient's arterial or venous system.

A ventricular assist device uses a blood pump or apparatus to augment or replace the function of the failing heart. Ventricular assist devices are designed to provide longer-term (weeks to months) support for patients with cardiac failure. These devices may serve as a bridge to recovery, to transplantation, or for permanent cardiac support. Unlike cardiopulmonary bypass and extracorporeal membrane oxygenation these devices do not incorporate a gas exchange system.

An intra-aortic balloon pump is a catheter mounted device that is used to provide short-term support in the setting of ventricular dysfunction or myocardial ischemia. It is inflated during ventricular diastole and deflated during ventricular systole. Thus, through "counterpulsation" it reduces systemic ventricular afterload and augments coronary artery perfusion.

	ECMO *	VAD **
Position	Extracorporeal	Para or extracorporeal
Pump	Roller or centripetal	Centripetal, pneumatic or vented electric
Oxygenator	Yes	No
Flow	Non-pulsatile	+/- pulsatile
Anticoagulation ***	ACT 180-240	ACT 140-180
In Line Dialysis Option	Yes	No
Respiratory Support	Yes	No
Cannulation	Neck vessels or mediastinal	Mediastinal

Table 4 - ECMO vs. VAD Support

* the use of ECMO support is generally limited to a period of several days
** the use of VAD support can be extended to periods of weeks or months
*** the use of heparin bonded circuit elements may allow periods of support with minimal systemic anticoagulation

329

SINGLE VENTRICLE (SV) POST-OPERATIVE MANAGEMENT

SV physiology encompasses a wide variety of anatomic lesions that have parallel circulations and complete mixing of systemic and pulmonary venous return.

Palliation for SV anatomy in most centers is performed via three stages with some variability in the initial stage procedure depending on degree of aortic outflow obstruction and amount of pulmonary blood flow. **Table 5** (pages 332-333) details the usual surgical interventions of patients with hypoplastic left heart syndrome (HLHS) and its variants.

Pages 306-307: Table 3 - Hypoplastic left heart syndrome surgical interventions

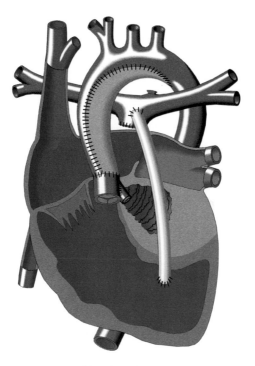

Above: Sano modification of Norwood Procedure for Hypoplastic Left Heart Syndrome

Table 5 - HYPOPLASTIC LEFT HEART SYNDROME SURGICAL INTERVENTIONS

TABLE 5	Stage I Norwood Procedure	Stage II Cavopulmonary Anastomosis Glenn or Hemi-Fontan Procedure	Stage III Fontan Completion
Goals	Unobstructed systemic blood flow (construction of a neo-aorta) Unobstructed PV return (atrial septectomy) Limited PBF without PA distortion (modified BTS or RV-PA conduit or a PA band)	Volume unloading of heart Creation of passive PBF	Pulmonary and systemic circulations in series
Post-operative Considerations	Total cardiac output and oxygen delivery is most important. Qp:Qs is predominately modulated by adjusting SVR. Avoid pulmonary venous desaturation with judicious use of PEEP and supplemental oxygen	Minimization of SVC-PA to atrial pressure gradient by • Early extubation • Elevation and midline position of head • Reduction of pulmonary edema (diuretics) • Monitor for pleural effusions • Commonly hypertensive (tx with nipride, nicardipine)	Arrhythmias • Post-operative period - sinus node dysfunction • Late - atrial arrhythmias • Ventricular dysfunction

	Stage I Norwood Procedure	Stage II Cavopulmonary Anastomosis Glenn or Hemi-Fontan Procedure	Stage III Fontan Completion
Low CO	• pure "pump failure" = inotropes • arrhythmia = restoration of sinus rhythm • Maldistribution of blood flow due to pulmonary overcirculation* or valvar regurgitation = afterload reduction		• Hypovolemia = volume • Increased PVR • Obstruction in systemic venous pathway
Hypoxemia-Etiologies	• low PV saturation → lung disease, pleural effusion or pneumothorax • low systemic venous saturation → anemia, low CO, or increased O_2 consumption • decreased Qp:Qs → shunt/conduit obstruction, severely elevated PVR, restrictive atrial septum (can treat acutely by raising the systemic BP)	• Elevated PVR • Veno-venous collaterals • Low PV saturation • SVC-PA connection obstruction	• low PV saturation→ lung disease, pleural effusion or pneumothorax • fenestration too large or a leak in lateral tunnel • decompressing veins • pulmonary AVMs

* pulmonary overcirculation due to arch obstruction needs to be addressed by surgical or catheter intervention

333

Table 6 - COMMONLY USED CICU VASOACTIVE MEDICATIONS

Drug	Mechanism	Inotropy	Chronotropy	SVR	PVR	Dose	Side Effects
Amiodarone	Class III antiarrhythmic, but with class IB, II and IV effects	$\leftrightarrow$ -	$\leftrightarrow$	$\leftrightarrow$	$\leftrightarrow$	Load 1-5 mg/kg Infusion 5-10 mcg/kg/min	Slows repolarization and AV conduction, prolongs QTc
Epinephrine	α_1 and $\beta_{1,2}$ agonist	+	+	$\leftarrow$	$\leftarrow$	Bolus 1-20 mcg/kg Infusion 0.05-2 mcg/kg/min	Hypertension, tachycardia, arrhythmias, myocardial necrosis
Dopamine	Dopaminergic-1, α_1 and β_1 agonist	$\leftrightarrow$	$\leftrightarrow$	$\leftarrow$	$\leftarrow$	Infusion-0.5-20 mcg/kg/min	Arrhythmias
Dobutamine	β_1 agonist	+	$\leftrightarrow$	$\leftrightarrow$	$\leftrightarrow$	Infusion 0.5-10 mcg/kg/min	Arrhythmias

Drug	Mechanism	Inotropy	Chronotropy	SVR	PVR	Dose	Side Effects
Isoproterenol	$\beta_{1,2}$ agonist	+	+	←	→	Infusion 0.05 mcg/kg/min – 1 mcg/kg/min	Arrhythmias
Milrinone	Phosphodiesterase 3 inhibitor	+	↕	→	→	Load 50 mcg/kg Infusion 0.25– 1.0 mcg/kg/min	Hypotension, thrombocytopenia
Norepinephrine	α_1 >>> β_1 agonist	+	+	←	←	Infusion 0.05-0.1 mcg/kg/min	Arrhythmias, Hypertension
Sildenafil	Phosphodiesterase 5 inhibitor	↕	↕	↕	→	PO/NG starting dose 0.25/ mg/kg Q6hr & titrate	Hypotension
Vasopression	V_{1a} agonist	↕	↕	←	↕	Infusion 0.0003-0.002 units/kg/min	Bradycardia, hyponatremia

Table 7 - COMMONLY USED CICU SEDATIVE/ANALGESIC MEDICATIONS

Class	Examples	Sedation	Analgesia	Other Effects	Notes
α-Adrenergic Agonist	Dexmedetomidine	+	-	Hypotension Bradycardia	Not recommended for >24 hr use
Barbiturate	Pentobarbital Phenobarbital	+	+	Anti-seizure	Minimal respiratory depression
Benzodiazepine	Midazolam Diazepam Lorazepam	+	-	Anti-seizure Amnesic Anxiolytic	
Dissociative	Ketamine	+	+	Amnestic	↑ secretions Emergence phenomenon
Narcotic	Fentanyl Morphine	+	+		Chest wall rigidity with rapid fentanyl administration Itching with morphine due to histamine release

REFERENCES

1. Shann, Kenneth G., Giacomuzzi, Carmen R., Harness, L., Myers, Gerard J., Paugh, Theron A., Mellas, Nicholas, Groom, R. C., Gomez, Daniel, Thuys, Clarke A., Charette, Kevin, Ojito, Jorge W., Tinius-Juliani, J., Calaritis, Christos, McRobb, C. M., Parpard, M., Chancy, Tom, Bacha, E., Cooper, D. S., Jacobs, Jeffrey P. , Likosky, Donald S., on behalf of the International Consortium for Evidence-Based Perfusion. Complications relating to perfusion and extracorporeal circulation associated with the treatment of patients with congenital cardiac disease: Consensus Definitions from the Multi-Societal Database Committee for Pediatric and Congenital Heart Disease. In: 2008 Supplement to Cardiology in the Young: Databases and The Assessment of Complications associated with The Treatment of Patients with Congenital Cardiac Disease, Prepared by: The Multi-Societal Database Committee for Pediatric and Congenital Heart Disease, Jeffrey P. Jacobs, MD (editor). Cardiology in the Young, Volume 18, Issue S2 (Suppl. 2), pp 206–214, December 9, 2008.

2. Shann, Kenneth G., Giacomuzzi, Carmen R., Jacobs, Jeffrey P., Myers, Gerard J., Paugh, Theron A., Mellas, Nicholas, Puis, Luc, Ojito, Jorge W., Gomez, Daniel, Olshove, Vincent, Fitzgerald, David C., Itoh, Hideshi, Brabant, Christopher, Thuys, Clarke A., Charette, Kevin, Calaritis, Christos, Parpard, Michael, Chancy, Tom, Baker, Robert A., Pourmoghadam, Kamal K., and Likosky, Donald S. Rationale and Use of Perfusion Variables in the 2010 Update of the Society of Thoracic Surgeons Congenital Heart Surgery Database. World Journal for Pediatric and Congenital Heart Surgery 2010 1: 34-43, April 2010.

3. Society of Thoracic Surgeons (STS) Congenital Heart Surgery Database Data Specifications Version 3.0 [http://www.sts.org/documents/pdf/CongenitalDataSpecificationsV3_0_20090904.pdf]. Accessed July 28, 2010.

CHAPTER 9.
INTRODUCTION TO ELECTROPHYSIOLOGY

By Jane E. Crosson, MD

Cardiac electrophysiology is the study of the cardiac conduction system and its abnormalities. The standard surface 12-lead electrocardiogram can provide a basic framework and understanding of the human conduction system, and is thus a useful everyday tool. More specialized testing such as an intracardiac electrophysiologic study can provide a more in-depth analysis and is crucial to the diagnosis and treatment of many arrhythmias.

THE ELECTROCARDIOGRAM

An electrocardiogram (ECG or EKG) is obtained by measuring the movement of electrical charges across the heart from a number of leads placed in various positions on the body, and displaying these wavefronts as vectors in two planes, the frontal and horizontal. The frontal plane (**Fig. 1**) is often referred to as Einthoven's triangle, and uses six orthogonal leads that display electrical activity in a superior-inferior and left-right orientation. The horizontal plane (**Fig. 2**) references electrodes positioned around the anterior and left chest.

Opposite:

> **Figure 1** - The frontal ECG axis -
> "Einthoven's triangle"

> **Figure 2** - ECG leads in the horizontal plane:
> 4VR; V1 through V6
>
> RV - right ventricle
> LV - left ventricle

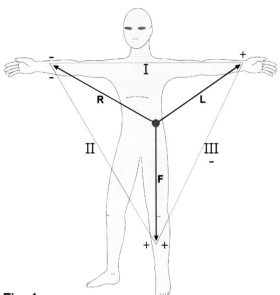

Fig. 1

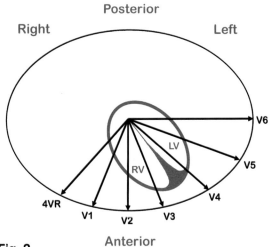

Fig. 2

341

Normal Conduction (Normal Sinus Rhythm)

The contraction of the heart muscle, which pumps blood to the lungs and body, is timed by the movement of electrical impulses. This movement is facilitated by specialized conduction system tissue. The Sinoatrial Node (SA) is the primary pacemaker of the heart (see **Fig. 3**), which spontaneously depolarizes, thus initiating each beat. Conduction then spreads through the atria to the Atrioventricular Node, normally the only electrical connection to the ventricles, and then through the muscles of the ventricles by means of the specialized His-Purkinje Fibers.

Vectors and Axes

The electrocardiogram cycle is divided into a series of three main phases (**Fig. 4**, page 345), the P wave (and PR interval), the QRS, and the T wave. These correspond to atrial depolarization (P), ventricular depolarization (QRS), and ventricular repolarization (T). These wavefront vectors as displayed on the ECG can provide valuable information about the heart's anatomy, size, and function. The mean vector is often called the axis. While P and T wave axes are important, the QRS axis in the frontal plane is especially valuable as a quick screen for heart disease. Abnormal QRS axes are commonly seen in congenital heart disease such as Atrioventricular Septal Defect (see pages 50-53), in which a superior (~240-300 degrees) axis is commonly seen, and in enlarged or hypertrophied hearts.

Opposite:

> **Figure 3** - Normal cardiac conduction system and electrocardiogram
>
> SA Node - Sinoatrial Node,
> AV Node - Atrioventricular Node

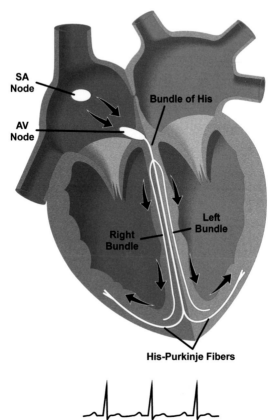

Fig. 3 - Normal Sinus Rhythm

343

ECG Intervals

The durations of specific intervals are also commonly analyzed ECG features. Major intervals include:

1. PR interval ('PRI' in **Figure 4**): time from onset of P wave to onset of QRS complex

2. QRS duration: total depolarization time for the ventricles.

3. QT interval: ('QTI' in **Figure 4**) total time from the onset of the QRS complex to the end of the T wave

Amplitude of ECG Signals

Atrial and ventricular hypertrophy can be assessed by the size of the P waves and QRS complexes, respectively. Criteria for right atrial enlargement are a P wave >2.5 mm tall in lead II, and for left atrial enlargement a notched or prolonged P wave >.1 sec (2.5 small boxes at normal ECG speed) in duration. Criteria for ventricular hypertrophy or enlargement are more complex, taking into account not only QRS size, but QRS and T wave axes.

Left Ventricular Hypertrophy

(LVH) occurs in patients with small right ventricles, as in tricuspid atresia, in left ventricular outflow obstruction, as in aortic stenosis, and in cardiomyopathies. There are several ECG markers that may be used to diagnose LVH, the most important being asymmetric T wave inversion in V5 and/or V6. However, it cannot be diagnosed if Bundle Branch Block is present.

Additional criteria are:

• R wave in V6 or S in V1 >98 percentile for age

• Deep but narrow Q waves in inferior leads (leads II, III, AVF)

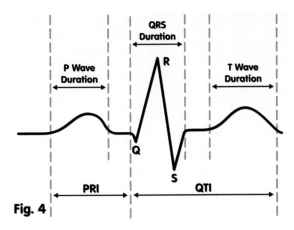

Figure 4. ECG Intervals

PRI - PR Interval, QTI - QT Interval

Right Ventricular Hypertrophy occurs in conditions that produce volume and/or pressure loads on the right ventricle, such as pulmonary stenosis, tetralogy of Fallot, pulmonary hypertension, and atrial septal defects. Criteria for RVH are more specific than for LVH.:

- qR pattern in V1, which is always abnormal

- Positive T wave in V1 between 1 week and teen

- R wave amplitude in V1 >98 percentile for age

- Deep S wave in V6 >98 percentile for age

- RSR' in V1: normal (incomplete RBBB), ASD or RV pressure overload

345

CONDUCTION DISTURBANCES

Bundle Branch Block is an abnormal prolongation of the QRS complex due to delay in conduction through a portion of the ventricular conduction system. Hypertrophy or ischemic changes can not be diagnosed if bundle branch block is present, because it masks the effect. (See page 343 for diagram of bundle branches.)

Opposite:

> **Figure 5A** - Left Bundle Branch Block (LBBB)
> Though generally uncommon in children, it can occur with left ventricular surgery or cardiomyopathy. Note delayed forces to the left.

> **Figure 5B** - Right Bundle Branch Block (RBBB)
> This is more common than left bundle branch block, especially after cardiac surgery such as repair of tetralogy of Fallot. Note delayed conduction to the right.

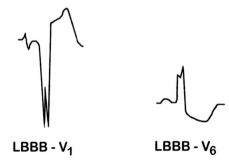

LBBB - V₁

LBBB - V₆

Fig. 5A

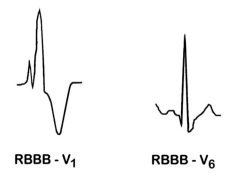

RBBB - V₁

RBBB - V₆

Fig. 5B

Pre-excitation

Pre-excitation is associated with an accessory connection between the atria and ventricles which allows early antegrade conduction to the ventricle. This will be discussed on page 354 under Accessory Connections.

Heart Block

- **First degree** heart block is a prolongation of the atrio-ventricular conduction time, producing a long PR interval. This may be seen after cardiac surgery or in rheumatic fever and is rarely a clinical concern.

- **Second degree** heart block results when some of the atrial beats are not conducted to the ventricle. In type 1 block, or "Wenkebach", there is progressive prolongation of the PR interval, eventually resulting in a loss of conduction to the ventricle. The pattern then repeats itself. If intermittent, this may be a normal finding, especially during sleep in otherwise healthy individuals. Type 2 block has a fixed PR interval, with a "dropped" QRS every 2nd or more beats (**Fig. 6, opposite**). This is more common post-surgically and in this setting may be a harbinger for complete block.

- **Third degree** (complete) heart block (**Fig. 7, opposite**) is diagnosed when no atrial beats are conducted to the ventricles. The ventricular rate is usually quite slow at 40-60 bpm. Patients are often symptomatic because of the inability to increase their heart rate with activity. Patients with complete heart block will usually require a pacemaker depending on their ventricular rate.

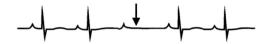

Fig. 6 - Second Degree Heart Block, Type 2
(Arrow indicates dropped QRS sequence.)

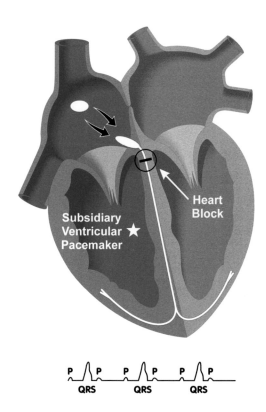

Fig. 7 - Complete Heart Block
(Smaller black arrows denote slowing of
impulse beyond heart block.)

349

ST-T Wave Abnormalities

The QT interval, measuring repolarization of the ventricles, is commonly corrected for heart rate using Bazett's formula ($QT/\sqrt{RR}$ intervals in seconds). It is prolonged in many electrolyte and metabolic disturbances, by medications, and in the long QT syndrome, a congenital abnormality in one of the cardiac ion channels. Patients with long QT syndrome or secondary prolonged QT are at risk for Torsade de Pointe, a characteristic form of ventricular tachycardia that is responsible for sudden death.

ST-T wave changes occur when there is inadequate oxygenation of the myocardium, such as in ischemia or frank myocardial infarction, and with inflammation of the pericardium in cardiomyopathies (**Fig. 8, opposite**).

ABNORMAL RHYTHMS

Rhythm disturbances (arrhythmias) can range from benign extra beats to life-threatening slow or fast rhythms. Arrhythmias often occur in otherwise normal hearts, but are more common in the setting of congenital heart disease and cardiomyopathy. There are three main types of arrhythmias: ectopic, or extra, beats such as premature ventricular contractions, slow rhythms (bradycardias), and fast rhythms (tachycardias). The latter two will be discussed further.

Bradycardias occur when 1) there is an abnormally slow sinus rate or 2) a lack of conduction of the sinus beats to the ventricles ("complete heart block"). Heart block will result in an atrial rate faster than the ventricular rate due to block around the AV node. This may be congenital or due to inadvertent surgical disruption of the conduction system during repair of congenital heart disease. The resulting ventricular escape rate is often quite slow, requiring a pacemaker.

Tachycardias may arise from cardiac tissue which has abnormal automaticity, via a re-entrant mechanism, or less commonly due to "triggered" activity. Tachycardia due to ab-

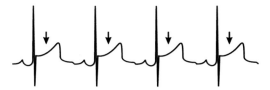

Fig. 8 - ST Elevation in V6
(Elevation indicated by arrows)

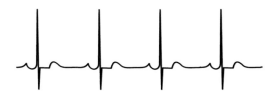

Normal tracing for comparison

351

normal automaticity occurs when an area of the heart depolarizes spontaneously at a rate exceeding the sinus rate. Both atrial and ventricular tachycardias can be due to abnormal automaticity.

Re-entrant mechanisms require an area of slow conduction, allowing a circle of electrical excitation to occur, which then perpetuates itself. In otherwise normal hearts this is often due to the presence of two pathways, each with slightly differing conduction and refractory periods (alpha and beta, see **A** in diagram, **opposite**).

The most classic example of this is supraventricular tachycardia (SVT) caused by an accessory AV pathway. An early beat (extrasystole) may expose the differing properties of these two pathways and can often initiate tachycardia. One pathway (often the 'slow' or beta pathway), may not conduct the premature beat at all (**B, opposite**). However, by the time the wavefront travels down the other 'fast' pathway, the distal end of the 'slow' pathway may be ready to conduct retrograde (but slowly), thus allowing the 'fast' pathway time to repolarize (**C, opposite**). When the wavefront reaches the beginning of the 'fast' pathway, the 'fast' pathway then depolarizes again, so that a 'round and round' pattern of depolarization is created.

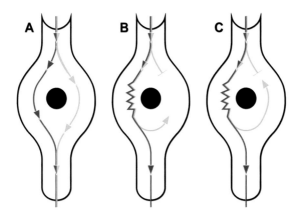

Figure 9. - Re-entrant Pathways and Tachycardia

A - alpha and beta (shown as left and right arrows) reen-
    trant pathways in myocardial tissue. Pathways conduct
    simultaneously; no re-entry circuit results.

B - Conduction though the right (beta) pathway is slow but
tissue is not refractory as is the left pathway.

C - repolarization of fast (alpha) pathway, re-entry circuit
    activated (see discussion on opposite page)

Arrhythmias - Accessory Pathways or Connections

An accessory connection is an extra electrical connection between atrial and ventricular tissue, in addition to the normal AV node conduction. It may not conduct all of the time, or it may conduct in only one direction. An accessory connection may be located anywhere along the AV groove, on either the left or right side of the heart. In this setting the tachycardia circuit usually involves normal antegrade conduction across the AV node and then retrograde conduction back to the atria through the pathway, as shown in the diagram (**Fig. 10, opposite**).

If an accessory connection does not support antegrade conduction (from the atria to the ventricles), and only conducts retrograde, it is called a **Concealed Accessory Connection**, as it will not be visible on a surface ECG while the heart is in normal sinus rhythm.

Wolff-Parkinson-White (WPW) Syndrome

If an accessory connection also allows antegrade conduction during normal sinus rhythm, there will be an area of the ventricular myocardium which will depolarize earlier than the usual conduction pathway through the AV node. This will manifest on the surface ECG as a **Delta Wave (Fig. 11, opposite)**. The delta wave occurs because of early activation of part of the ventricle by the pathway. The QRS appears wider due to necessarily slower conduction cell-to-cell through the ventricular tissue, rather than over the rapidly conducting His-Purkinje system. In the setting of SVT, this pattern is called "Wolff-Parkinson-White syndrome (WPW)."

Opposite:

> **Figure 10** - Internal diagram of heart showing an accessory atrioventricular connection (indicated by arrow)

> **Figure 11** - Diagram of ECG showing the Delta Wave, characteristic of WPW

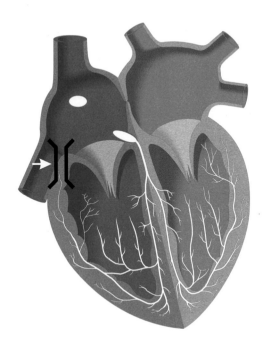

Fig. 10 - Accessory Atrioventricular Connection

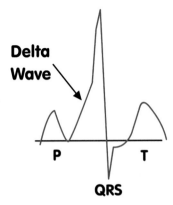

Fig. 11 - Delta Wave

355

WPW is also called "manifest pre-excitation" as the abnormality can be seen on the normal sinus rhythm ECG and "pre-excites" part of the ventricle. Only 50% of accessory connections are due to WPW, but WPW always requires an accessory connection. WPW can be more dangerous than a concealed AV connection, due to the possibility of rapid antegrade conduction of atrial arrhythmias through the pathway triggering ventricular fibrillation.

WPW Syndrome is pre-excitation caused by an anomalous A-V conduction pathway and is characterized by the following:

1) Short PR interval
2) Delta wave
3) Wide QRS

Opposite:

Figure 12 - SVT: AVNT (atrioventricular reciprocating tachycardia, also called ORT)

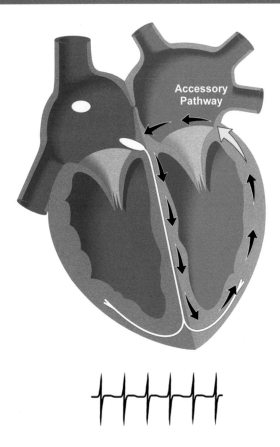

Fig. 12

357

The tachycardia described on pages 350 and 352, where the AV node is the antegrade limb of the tachycardia and an accessory connection is the retrograde limb, is commonly known by the non-specific term "supraventricular tachycardia" (SVT). It is more precisely called "orthodromic reciprocating tachycardia" (ORT), or atrioventricular reciprocating tachycardia" (AVNT), which describes the back and forth movement between the atria and ventricles involved in maintaining the tachycardia circuit. Whether the involved pathway is "manifest" (WPW) or "concealed", the ECG during tachycardia will look the same, as both conduct retrograde to the atria. Heart rates typically range from 220 bpm to 300 bpm.

Atrial Flutter or "atrial re-entry tachycardia" is a very common re-entry tachycardia originating from the atria. This tachycardia is most commonly found in a natural area of slow conduction in the inferior portion of the right atrium, or is due to an area of scar tissue in the atria. In this tachycardia, shown in **Fig. 13, opposite**, the ventricle is a 'bystander', passively receiving rapid impulses from the atria. The atrial rate is commonly 300 with two or three atrial beats for every ventricular response (2:1 or 3:1 conduction), as the AV node provides some protection against rapid conduction to the ventricle.

Ventricular tachycardia is less common in children than in adults, where it is usually secondary to ischemic heart disease. Ventricular tachycardia (**Fig. 14, opposite**) in children is often secondary to congenital heart disease or cardiomyopathy, but may be seen in otherwise normal hearts. Ventricular tachycardia is often a very unstable rhythm and requires immediate treatment.

Opposite:

> **Figure 13** - Atrial Flutter with 3:1 conduction - heart diagram and ECG

> **Figure 14** - Ventricular Tachycardia - ECG

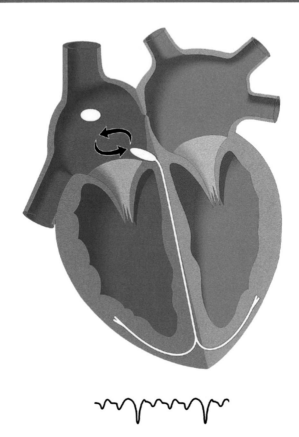

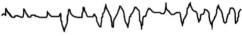

Fig. 13 - Atrial Flutter

Fig. 14 - Ventricular Tachycardia

EVALUATION OF ARRHYTHMIAS

A **Holter monitor** is a 24 or 48 hour constant recording of the patient's heart beat. ECG leads are fixed to the body and attached to a small recording device. This is useful for patients with frequent symptoms or occult arrhythmias, or to evaluate the need for a pacemaker in a patient with congenital heart block.

A **transient event recorder** is more useful in patients with less frequent events. "Looping" monitors stay attached at all times and can be programmed to record the rhythm at pre-set high or low heart rates, and/or triggered by the patient or caregiver. Since these devices are capable of storing data in memory, even short-lived or occult arrhythmias can be recorded. For episodes with longer duration, "non-looping" recorders are more convenient. These can be carried by the patient and very quickly attached at the onset of symptoms. Both of these devices will store recordings until they can be downloaded over a telephone connection.

Implantable monitors are less widely used in children. These small, wireless recording devices are implanted under the skin, similar to pacemaker placement. Although more invasive, they can be actively used for months in patients with infrequent but severe symptoms.

An **electrophysiology study** is a catheter-based procedure performed to determine the mechanism of tachycardia and the location of arrhythmia circuits such as accessory pathways. Multiple electrode catheters are placed in the heart to record the electrical activity from the atria, ventricles, and AV node, and can be used to stimulate the heart into the arrhythmia to be studied. (Catheter positions shown in **Fig. 15, opposite.**)

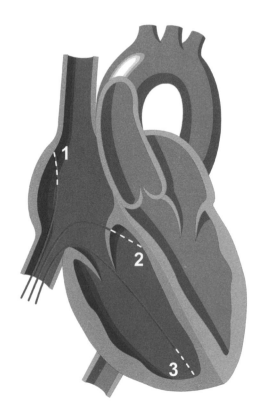

Fig. 15

Above: Electrode catheters in the (**1**) - right atrium; (**2**) - "His" position); and (**3**) - right ventricle

TREATMENT OF ARRHYTHMIAS

Medications may be used alone or in conjunction with procedures to restore normal cardiac activity. They are used primarily for short-term treatment or when the arrhythmia cannot be easily and safely treated with more definitive measures. (See Chapter 10, **Common Cardiac Pharmaceuticals**, for information on specific medications.)

Electrical cardioversion is a procedure in which an electrical charge is introduced into the heart, "resetting" its rhythm and allowing the heart's normal timing mechanism to reassert itself. This is usually performed by placing patches on the anesthetized patient's chest, through which a direct current charge is delivered.

If an amenable tachycardia circuit is identified during an electrophysiology study, an **ablation procedure** (see **Fig. 16**, **opposite**) can be performed to eliminate the abnormal electrical pathways using a catheter within the heart. Current ablation techniques use radio-frequency or cryotherapy to produce thermal damage to the tissue. Surgical ablation techniques are an option for patients who are undergoing other cardiac surgery, or when catheter ablation has failed.

Opposite:

> **Figure 16** - An ablation procedure. The catheter is directed to the location on the AV groove determined to be the site of the abnormal electrical pathway. The pathway is eliminated via thermal damage to the tissue.

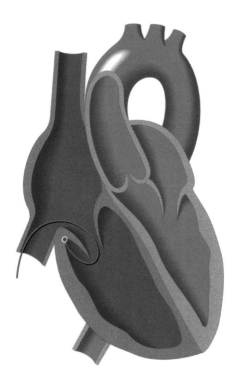

Fig. 16

363

Bradycardias are often treated by implanting a **pacemaker** to re-establish a more normal rate and rhythm. A battery and control box, termed the "generator", is placed under the skin, and pacemaker leads are attached to the heart either through the veins ("transvenous") or from the outside of the heart ("epicardial"). (See diagram of pacemaker system **opposite**.)

In some patients with congenital heart disease, the leads often cannot be placed inside the heart due to the presence of prosthetic valves, or a concern about thromboembolus in the setting of a single ventricle. Infants and young children do not have large enough veins to accommodate transvenous systems. In these cases, epicardial leads are placed surgically.

A specialized form of the pacemaker, the **implantable cardioverter-defibrillator (ICD)**, can be programmed to automatically pace and/or shock the heart back into a normal rhythm if a tachycardia is detected. The usual indication for an ICD is a concern about ventricular tachycardia.

Opposite:

> **Figure 17** - Dual chamber pacing system (atrial and ventricular leads) with generator (see arrow) below left clavicle and transvenous leads in the right atrium and right ventricle

REFERENCES

Davignon A, et al. Normal ECG standards for infants and children. *Pediatric Cardiology*, 1979;1:123-131.

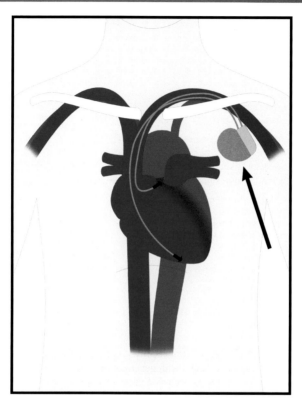

Fig. 17

365

CHAPTER 10.
COMMON CARDIAC PHARMACEUTICALS

By Marcia L. Buck, PharmD

See following tables for alphabetical listing of medications, with information under the following categories:

> Drug Name
> Class and Mechanism of Action
> Dosing Guidelines
> Pharmacokinetics
> Adverse Effects
> Notes

Notes and References - 412

Please note: This information is intended as a quick reference and is not a complete source of drug information. Readers are encouraged to consult the prescribing information provided by the drug manufacturer for additional guidance. The doses listed are based on current literature, and the reader is advised that the author and editors cannot be responsible for the continued currency of this information or any errors from the application of this information.

Common Cardiac Pharmaceuticals

CARDIAC MEDICATIONS FOR INFANTS AND CHILDREN (See note 1, page 412.)

DRUG NAME	CLASS & MECHANISM OF ACTION	DOSING GUIDELINES	PHARMACOKINETICS	ADVERSE EFFECTS	NOTES
Adenosine	Antiarrhythmic; slows conduction through the AV node, interrupting re-entry pathways	Pediatrics: 0.1-0.3 mg/kg/dose rapid IV push Adult dose: 6 mg, if no response, increase to max dose of 12 mg	$T_{1/2}$ < 10 sec Removed from circulation by vascular endothelial cells and erythrocytes	Bronchospasm, flushing, chest pain, headache, nausea, metallic taste	Larger doses may be needed in patients receiving methylxanthines (aminophylline, theophylline, or caffeine)
Alprostadil	Prostaglandin E_1 (PGE_1) Dilates ductus arteriosus to maintain fetal circulation pattern	0.01 to 0.1 mcg/kg/min IV infusion; titrate to lowest effective dose to minimize apnea	$T_{1/2}$ = 5-10 min Metabolized in lungs	Apnea, hypotension, fever, seizures, electrolyte imbalances, diarrhea Long-term: gastric outlet obstruction, cortical hyperostosis	Compatible with parenteral nutrition solution To reduce risk of apnea, treat with aminophylline or caffeine.

Common Cardiac Pharmaceuticals

Ambrisentan	Selective ETA endothelin receptor antagonist used to treat pulmonary hypertension	Adults: initial dose 5 mg PO once daily, increase to 10 mg once daily if needed Pediatric dosing not yet established	$T_{1/2}$ = 15 hrs in adults Hepatic metabolism via multiple pathways including CYP3A4 and CYP2C19	Hepatic dysfunction, headache, dizziness, dyspnea, flushing, edema, constipation	Available only in tablet form through a limited distribution program Significant risk for birth defects if taken during pregnancy
Amiodarone	Class III antiarrhythmic; prolongs the action potential and refractory period; decreases AV conduction and sinus node function (continued)	Loading dose: 5 mg/kg IV over 1 hr or as five 1 mg/kg aliquots, each given over 5 - 10 min Infusion: 5 - 15 mcg/kg/min Oral loading dose: 10 to 15 mg/kg/day for 4-14 days	$T_{1/2}$ = 20 to 50 days Extensive accumulation with repeated dosing; Metabolized by hepatic and GI cytochrome P450 3A3/4	Arrhythmias, bradycardia, hypotension, ataxia, dizziness, behavioral changes, nausea, anorexia, thrombocytopenia, phlebitis, tremor, corneal microdeposits, (continued on next page)	Leaches DEHP from soft plastics. Numerous drug interactions, including inhibition of digoxin clearance (reduce digoxin dose by approximately 50%) (continued on next page)

Common Cardiac Pharmaceuticals

DRUG NAME	CLASS & MECHANISM OF ACTION	DOSING GUIDELINES	PHARMACO-KINETICS	ADVERSE EFFECTS	NOTES
Amiodarone (continued)		(Pediatrics, continued) Maintenance: 2.5 to 5 mg/kg/day PO divided and given BID

Adults: ACLS doses for pulseless VT/VF: 300 mg IV/IO; repeat with another 150 mg if needed | | (continued) interstitial pneumonitis, pulmonary fibrosis, hepatotoxicity, altered thyroid function, altered skin color, photosensitivity | (continued) May act as a vaso-dilator and nega-tive inotrope Available in tablet form; can be pre-pared as an oral liquid (see references) |
| Amlodipine | Dihydropyri-dine calcium channel blocker (reduces SVR with little effect on myo-cardium) | Pediatrics: 0.05 to 0.2 mg/kg/day PO QD

Adults: 2.5 - 5 mg/day (max 10 mg/day) | $T_{1/2}$ = 30-50 hrs

Hepatic metabolism | Hypotension, edema, headache, dizziness, flushing, tachycardia, weakness, cramps, nau-sea, rash, angioedema, sexual dysfunction, gynecomastia, gingival hyperplasia (rare) | Available in tablet form; can be pre-pared as an oral liquid (see references) |

Common Cardiac Pharmaceuticals

		Weight	Daily Dose (using 81 mg tab)			
Aspirin	Analgesic, antipyretic, antiplatelet agent Blocks prostaglandin synthetase, preventing formation of the platelet-aggregating substance thromboxane A_2	2-6 kg 7-13 kg 14-30 kg 31-40 kg > 40 kg	¼ tablet ½ tablet 1 tablet 1 ½ tablet 2 tablets or 1 tablet (81 or 325 mg)	$T_{1/2}$ = 15-20 min Hepatic metabolism Serum concentration goal: 100 mcg/ml (trough) Serum concentration monitoring is not necessary for most patients	GI upset, gastric bleeding, hemorrhage, tinnitus, interstitial nephritis, hepatotoxicity	The table at left is based on the usual maintenance dose after shunt placement, Fontan, or for Kawasaki Syndrome: 3-5 mg/kg/day For patients with mechanical valves unable to tolerate warfarin, usual dose 6-20 mg/kg/day, up to 325 mg max

Common Cardiac Pharmaceuticals

DRUG NAME	CLASS & MECHANISM OF ACTION	DOSING GUIDELINES	PHARMACOKI-NETICS	ADVERSE EFFECTS	NOTES
Atenolol	β_1- adrenergic blocking agent; antihypertensive and Class II antiarrhythmic	Pediatrics: 1-2 mg/kg/day PO given daily or divided and given every 12 hrs Adults: 25-50 mg/day (max 100 mg/day)	$T_{1/2}$ = 3-7 hrs Primarily renal elimination	Hypotension, bradycardia, headache, dizziness, confusion, nausea, bronchoconstriction	**Adjust dose in patients with renal dysfunction.** Available in tablet form; can be prepared as an oral liquid (see references)
Atropine	Inhibits the action of acetylcholine at parasympathetic sites; increases heart rate and cardiac output	0.02 mg/kg, may repeat in 5 min (max dose 0.5 mg in children, 1 mg in adolescents/adults)	$T_{1/2}$ = 3-10 hrs in children < 2 years, 1-3 hrs in children > 2 years. Hepatic metabolism and renal elimination as unchanged drug	Arrhythmias, headache, dizziness, confusion, hyperpyrexia, dry mouth, decreased GI motility, urinary retention, blurred vision, mydriasis, tachypnea, pulmonary edema	Paradoxical bradycardia may be seen with doses < 0.1 mg

Common Cardiac Pharmaceuticals

Benazepril	ACE inhibitor	Children > 6 years: Initial: 0.2 mg/kg PO QD; up to 0.6 mg/kg/day or 40 mg/day Adults: initial dose 10 mg PO QD, usual maintenance 20-40 mg/day (max 80 mg/day)	$T_{1/2}$ = 5 hrs in children, 22 hrs in adults Converted to active benazeprilat in the liver; further metabolized to inactive compounds	Hypotension, hypersensitivity reactions, angioedema, hyperkalemia, neutropenia, agranulocytosis, hepatic dysfunction (rare), proteinuria, cough, altered taste	Available in tablet form; can be prepared as an oral liquid (see Lotensin® prescribing information/package insert)
Bosentan	ET_a and ET_A endothelin receptor antagonist; used to treat pulmonary hypertension	Children 10-20 kg: 31.25 mg PO BID Children > 20 kg and Adults: 62.5 mg PO BID (approximately 1.5-3 mg/kg/day), increase to 125 mg PO BID after 1 month if serum transaminases remain within normal limits	$T_{1/2}$ = 4-6 hrs Hepatic metabolism via cytochrome P450 2C9 and 3A4	Hepatic dysfunction, headache, dizziness, cough, dyspnea, flushing, edema	Available in tablet form through a limited distribution program directly from the manufacturer; can be prepared as on oral liquid (see references) Significant risk for birth defects if taken during pregnancy

373

DRUG NAME	CLASS & MECHANISM OF ACTION	DOSING GUIDELINES	PHARMACO-KINETICS	ADVERSE EFFECTS	NOTES
Bumetanide	Loop diuretic; inhibits sodium and chloride reabsorption in the ascending loop of Henle and distal renal tubule	Pediatrics: 0.015 - 0.1 mg/kg/ dose IV every 6 to 24 hours (max 10 mg/day) 0.015 - 0.1 mg/kg/ dose PO QD-QID (max 10 mg/day) Adults: 0.5-2 mg IV/PO once daily (max 10 mg/day)	$T_{1/2}$ = 6 hrs in neonates; 2.5 hrs in infants < 2 months; 1.5 hrs in older infants to adults. Metabolized and also excreted unchanged in the urine.	Hypotension, ↓K, Na, Ca, Mg, and Cl, hyperglycemia, headache, dizziness, weakness, diarrhea, rash, photosensitivity, nephrocalcinosis, ototoxicity, agranulocytosis	
Calcium chloride	Increases cardiac contractility	Pediatrics: 10 - 20 mg/kg/dose IV every 4-6 hrs (max 1 gram/dose) Adults: 1 gram IV every 6 hrs		Bradydysrhythmias, hypotension, hypercalcemia, hypermagnesemia, hyperchloremic acidosis, coma, emesis, constipation	Not compatible with sodium bicarbonate; Administer centrally; extravasation may cause necrosis (use hyaluronidase to minimize damage).

Common Cardiac Pharmaceuticals

Drug	Class	Dose	Pharmacokinetics	Adverse Effects	Comments
Calcium gluconate	Increases cardiac contractility	Pediatrics: 50 - 100 mg/kg/dose IV every 4-6 hrs (max 3 gram/dose) Adults: 1 gram IV every 6 hrs (max 3 gram/dose)		Bradydysrhythmias, hypotension, hypercalcemia, hypermagnesemia, hyperchloremic acidosis, coma, emesis, constipation	Not compatible with sodium bicarbonate; Administer centrally whenever possible; extravasation may cause necrosis (use hyaluronidase to minimize damage).
Captopril	ACE inhibitor	Initial dose: Infants: 0.01-0.1 mg/kg/dose PO BID-QID Children: 0.3-0.5 mg/kg/dose PO given BID-QID, up to 6 mg/kg/day Adults: 12.5-25 mg PO BID-TID up to 450 mg/day	$T_{1/2}$ = 1-2 hrs (prolonged in infants with cardiac failure) Renal elimination	Hypotension, tachycardia, headache, dizziness, rash, angioedema, hyperkalemia, neutropenia, agranulocytosis, hepatic dysfunction (rare), proteinuria, cough, altered taste	**Adjust dose in patients with renal dysfunction.** Long-term use associated with zinc deficiency, which may lead to altered taste. Available in tablet form; can be prepared as an oral liquid (see references)

Common Cardiac Pharmaceuticals

DRUG NAME	CLASS & MECHANISM OF ACTION	DOSING GUIDELINES	PHARMACOKINETICS	ADVERSE EFFECTS	NOTES
Carvedilol	Nonselective β-blocker with α$_1$ adrenergic blocking properties providing additional vasodilation	Pediatrics: 0.01-0.2 mg/kg/day PO divided and given BID or TID; titrate up to 0.7 mg/kg/day as needed Adults: 3.125-6.25 mg PO BID	T$_{1/2}$ = 2-3 hrs (5 hrs in adults) Hepatic metabolism	Hypotension, edema, worsening of heart failure, bradycardia, dizziness, headache, bronchospasm, rash, hypersensitivity reactions, diarrhea, renal toxicity or hepatotoxicity (rare)	Available in tablet form; can be prepared as an oral liquid (see references)
Chloral hydrate	Sedative (no analgesic properties) Used for nonpainful procedures of long duration	Neonates: 25 mg/kg/dose Children: 50-100 mg/kg/dose PO or PR (max 2 grams) single dose for procedural sedation	Onset: 1/2-1 hr Duration: 4-9 hrs T$_{1/2}$ = 10 hrs Hepatic metabolism to active trichloroethanol metabolite	CNS and respiratory depression, arrhythmias (rare), paradoxical agitation, urticaria	Bitter taste Potential for prolonged effect with repeat dosing

Common Cardiac Pharmaceuticals

Chlorothiazide	Thiazide diuretic Inhibits Na+ reabsorption in the distal tubule	Pediatrics: 4-20 mg/kg/day as continuous infusion or divided and given every 12 hrs IV; 20-40 mg/kg/day PO divided and given BID (max 1 gram/day) Adults: 500-1 gram PO once or twice daily	$T_{1/2}$ = 1-2 hrs (adults) Excreted unchanged in the urine	Hypotension, electrolyte imbalances, headache, dizziness, weakness, diarrhea, rash, photosensitivity	Can be infused with furosemide. Available as injection, tablet, and 50 mg/ml oral liquid.
Clonidine	α_2 - adrenergic agonist in CNS; reduces sympathetic tone and produces vasodilation	Pediatrics: 5-10 mcg/kg/day PO divided and given BID-TID (max 0.9 mg/day) Adults: 0.1 mg PO BID (max 2.4 mg/day)	$T_{1/2}$ = 8-12 hrs Hepatic metabolism and renal excretion	Hypotension, bradycardia, sedation, dizziness, rash, edema, constipation, rebound hypertension with abrupt withdrawal	Available in tablet form; can be prepared as an oral liquid (see references). Transdermal patch 0.1, 0.2, or 0.3 mg/day (changed weekly)

Common Cardiac Pharmaceuticals

DRUG NAME	CLASS & MECHANISM OF ACTION	DOSING GUIDELINES	PHARMACOKINETICS	ADVERSE EFFECTS	NOTES
Clopidogrel	Inhibits platelet aggregation; Active metabolite modifies the P2Y$_{12}$ platelet receptor, preventing binding of ADP	Neonates and infants < 24 months: 0.2 mg/kg PO once daily Children: 1 mg/kg PO once daily Adults: 300 mg or 600 mg PO loading dose, followed by 75 mg PO daily	$T_{1/2}$ = 8 hrs (primary inactive metabolite) Hepatic metabolism	Hemorrhage, hypertension, edema, headache, dizziness, rash, GI upset, arthralgias, hypercholesterolemia	Available in tablet form; can be prepared as an oral liquid (see references). Do not administer with proton pump inhibitors such as omeprazole.
Codeine	Opioid sedative/analgesic, antitussive	Pediatrics: 0.5-1 mg/kg/dose PO every 4-6 hrs (max 60 mg per dose)	Onset: 30-60 minutes Duration: 4-6 hrs $T_{1/2}$ =2-4 hrs Hepatic metabolism to morphine and inactive compounds	CNS and respiratory depression, hypotension, bradycardia, emesis, pruritus, urinary retention	*IV use not recommended due to large amount of histamine released causing hypotension. Reversal agent: naloxone (Narcan®) 5-10 mcg/kg/dose every 2-3 min (See note #2.)

Digoxin	Inotrope; antiarrhythmic Inhibits Na/K movement across membranes, increasing intracellular calcium	**Total Digitalizing Dose:** Pediatrics: 8-20 mcg/kg IV (divided into three doses) Maintenance: 2-10 mcg/kg/day PO/IV given once daily or divided and given BID Adults: 0.125 mg -0.250 mg PO once daily	$T_{1/2}$ = 20-40 hrs 50-70% excreted unchanged in urine	Arrhythmias (incl. heart block), dizziness, sedation, hyperkalemia, emesis, vision changes, neuralgias, diarrhea	Therapeutic range: 0.8 to 2 ng/mL Check for drug interactions. Multiple dosage forms available, including 50 mcg/mL oral liquid.
Diltiazem	Calcium channel blocker; antihypertensive Relaxes muscle by inhibition of calcium influx during depolarization	Pediatrics: 1-2 mg/kg/day PO divided and given TID or QID Adults: 180-480 mg/day (depending on preparation chosen)	$T_{1/2}$ = 3-5 hrs in adults Hepatic metabolism; large first-pass effect; active metabolite desacetyldiltiazem	Arrhythmias, hypotension, headache dizziness, insomnia, rash, photosensitivity, nausea, vomiting, weakness, rare leukopenia or thrombocytopenia, rare exfoliative dermatitis	*IV use not recommended. Numerous drug interactions. May be used to increase cyclosporine concentrations. Available in tablet form; can be prepared as an oral liquid (see references).

Common Cardiac Pharmaceuticals

DRUG NAME	CLASS & MECHANISM OF ACTION	DOSING GUIDELINES	PHARMACO-KINETICS	ADVERSE EFFECTS	NOTES
Diphenhydr-amine	Antihistamine; Sedative (no analgesic properties); use for nonpainful procedures	Pediatrics: 1-2 mg/kg/dose PO, IM, or IV Adults: 25-50 mg PO, IM, or IV every 6 hours max 300 mg/day	Onset: 1/2-1 hr Duration: 4-7 hrs $T_{1/2}$ = 2-8 hrs Hepatic metabolism with extensive first-pass effect	Hypotension, dizziness, emesis, dry mucous membranes, urinary retention, blurred vision, tremor; paradoxical agitation	
Dipyridamole	Antiplatelet agent; Inhibits the activity of adenosine deaminase and phosphodiesterase, resulting in inhibition of platelet aggregation	Pediatrics: 2-5 mg/kg/day PO divided and given TID, in combination with low-dose warfarin and/or aspirin Adults: 75-100 mg PO TID or QID	$T_{1/2}$ = 10-12 hrs Hepatic metabolism	Flushing, syncope, dizziness, headache, rash, nausea, vomiting, weakness, rare hepatotoxicity	Available in tablet form; can be prepared as an oral liquid (see references).

Dobutamine	Synthetic catecholamine β₁ agonist; Inotrope	Pediatrics: 2-20 mcg/kg/min IV (doses up to 40 mcg/kg/min have been used)	$T_{1/2}$ = 2 min Metabolized throughout body by monoamine oxidase and catechol-O-methyl-transferase	Arrhythmias, hypertension, emesis, dyspnea	Not compatible with alkaline solutions (e.g. sodium bicarbonate). Administer centrally; extravasation risk. Administer phentolamine as soon as possible after extravasation.
Dofetilide	Class III antiarrhythmic; blocks I_{Kr} ion channel, resulting in delayed repolarization	Adults: 500 mcg PO BID Reduce dose in patients with renal dysfunction Pediatric dosing not yet established	$T_{1/2}$ = 10 hrs in adults 80% renal excretion, primarily as unchanged drug; small amounts metabolized by CYP3A4	Arrhythmias, hypertension, chest pain, headache, dizziness, nausea	Treatment must be initiated with continuous ECG monitoring and personnel able to manage serious ventricular arrhythmias for a minimum of 3 days. Additive effect with other drugs that prolong the QT interval

Common Cardiac Pharmaceuticals

DRUG NAME	CLASS & MECHANISM OF ACTION	DOSING GUIDELINES	PHARMACO-KINETICS	ADVERSE EFFECTS	NOTES
Dopamine	Endogenous catechol-amine; β₁ agonist, α agonist; Inotrope and vasopressor	Dopaminergic effects: 1-5 mcg/kg/min IV β₁ effects: 5-15 mcg/kg/min IV α effects: 15-20 mcg/kg/min IV * high interpatient variability	$T_{1/2}$ = 2 min Metabolized throughout body by monoamine oxidase and catechol-O-methyltransferase to norepinephrine and inactive metabolites	Arrhythmias, hypertension, emesis, dyspnea, dilated pupils	Not compatible with alkaline solutions (e.g. sodium bicarbonate). Administer centrally; extravasation risk. Administer phentolamine as soon as possible after extravasation.

Common Cardiac Pharmaceuticals

Drug	Class	Dose	Pharmacokinetics	Side Effects	Notes
Enalapril	ACE inhibitor	Pediatrics: 0.1-0.5 mg/kg/day PO given QD/BID Adults: 2.5-5 mg/day (max 40 mg/day)	$T_{1/2}$ = 2-3 hrs (up to 10 hrs in premature infants); Enalapril (a prodrug) is converted to active enalaprilat in the liver.	Hypotension, dizziness, headache, rash, angioedema, hypoglycemia, hyperkalemia, anemia, neutropenia, hepatic or renal dysfunction (rare)	**Adjust dose in patients with renal dysfunction.** Available in tablet form; can be prepared as an oral liquid (see Vasotec® prescribing information package insert).
Enalaprilat	ACE inhibitor	Pediatrics: 5 to 10 mcg/kg/ dose IV every 8 to 24 hours Adults: 0.625-1.25 mg IV every 6 hours	$T_{1/2}$ = 6-10 hours Excreted unchanged in urine	Hypotension, dizziness, headache, rash, angioedema, hypoglycemia, hyperkalemia, anemia, neutropenia, hepatic or renal dysfunction (rare)	

DRUG NAME	CLASS & MECHANISM OF ACTION	DOSING GUIDELINES	PHARMACO-KINETICS	ADVERSE EFFECTS	NOTES
Enoxaparin	Anticoagulant; A low-molecular-weight heparin; Potentiates the action of anti-thrombin III; inactivates factor Xa and to a lesser degree, factor IIa (thrombin)	Age < 2 months; Prophylaxis 0.75 mg/kg every 12 hrs SQ Treatment 1.5 mg/kg every 12 hrs SQ > 2 months; Prophylaxis 0.5 mg/kg every 12 hrs SQ Treatment 1 mg/kg every 12 hrs SQ Reduce interval to once daily for patients with severe renal dysfunction	Antifactor-Xa level goal: 0.5-1 units/ml Obtain level 4 hrs post-dose	Hemorrhage, thrombo-cytopenia, injection site reactions, edema, fever, hematuria	Anti-Xa Adjustment < 0.35 ----- Increase dose by 25% 0.35-0.49 -- Increase dose by 10% 0.5-1 ----- No change 1.1-1.5 ----- Decrease dose by 20% 1.6-2 ----- Hold for 3 hrs, then decrease dose by 30% > 2 ----- Hold until < 0.5 then restart after 40% decrease

Common Cardiac Pharmaceuticals

Epinephrine	Endogenous catecholamine; β_1 agonist α agonist; Inotrope and vasopressor	0.01 to 1 mcg/kg/min IV Bolus: 0.01 mg/kg IV (max 1 mg)	$T_{1/2}$ = 1-2 min Metabolized throughout body by monoamine oxidase and catechol-O-methyltransferase to norepinephrine	Arrhythmias, hypertension, emesis, weakness, urinary retention	Not compatible with alkaline solutions (e.g. sodium bicarbonate). Administer centrally; extravasation risk. Administer phentolamine as soon as possible after extravasation.
Epoprostenol	Prostacyclin (PGI_2) Pulmonary vasodilator	Initiate at 1 to 2 ng/kg/min IV, titrate every 15 min to optimal effect	$T_{1/2}$ < 6 min Hydrolyzed at neutral pH in blood	Hypotension, emesis, headache, chest pain, flushing, jaw pain, anxiety, dyspnea, ↑heart rate	Can also be administered by inhalation, with doses ranging from 3 to 100 ng/kg/min. Sudden discontinuation may lead to rebound pulmonary hypertension.

DRUG NAME	CLASS & MECHANISM OF ACTION	DOSING GUIDELINES	PHARMACOKI-NETICS	ADVERSE EFFECTS	NOTES
Esmolol	β_1- adrenergic blocking agent; antihypertensive and Class II antiarrhythmic	Loading dose: 100-500 mcg/kg IV over 1 min Infusion: 50 -1000 mcg/kg/min usual rate 500 mcg/kg/min	$T_{1/2}$ = 2-4 min Metabolized by blood esterases	Hypotension, bradycardia, headache, dizziness, nausea, confusion, diaphoresis, bronchoconstriction	Cardioselectivity is lost at higher doses.
Fentanyl	Opioid sedative/analgesic	Pediatrics: Intermittent dose: 1-3 mcg/kg/dose IV/IM may repeat in 30-60 min Infusion: 1-3 mcg/kg/hr Adults: 25-50 mcg/dose IV or IM	Onset: 1 - 3 min duration: 30 min-2 hrs $T_{1/2}$ = 2-4 hrs Hepatic metabolism	CNS and respiratory depression, hypotension, bradycardia, emesis, pruritus, urinary retention Muscle rigidity with rapid IV bolus.	**If using with a benzodiazepine: decrease dose by 25-50% to avoid respiratory depression.** Less cardiovascular effects than morphine Reversal agent: naloxone (Narcan®) 5-10 mcg/kg/dose every 2-3 min (See note #2.)

			Decrease dose by 25 to 50% in children with severe renal dysfunction.
Flecainide	Class IC antiarrhythmic; slows conduction by altering ion transport across cell membranes	Pediatrics: 1-3 mg/kg/day PO divided and given TID; up to 8 mg/kg/day Adults: initial dose 100 mg PO BID, increase as needed to max dose 400 mg/day	$T_{1/2}$ = 20 hrs in neonates, 11-12 hrs in infants, 8 hrs in children Hepatic metabolism	Arrhythmias, headache, fatigue, rash, nausea, blood dyscrasias, hepatic dysfunction, dyspnea, tremor	Administration with milk or formula may decrease absorption. Available in tablet form; can be prepared as an oral liquid (see references).
Furosemide	Loop diuretic Inhibits sodium and chloride reabsorption in the ascending loop of Henle and distal renal tubule	Pediatrics: 1-2 mg/kg/dose IV or PO every 6-24 hrs or 0.05-0.4 mg/kg/hr infusion Adults: 20-40 mg IV or PO every 6-24 hours	$T_{1/2}$ = 30 min-1 hr Excreted primarily unchanged in the urine.	Hypotension, ↓ K, Na, Ca, Mg, and Cl, hyperglycemia, headache, dizziness, weakness, diarrhea, rash, photosensitivity, neprocalcinosis, ototoxicity, agranulocytosis	Maximum rate of IV bolus administration 0.5 mg/kg/min

DRUG NAME	CLASS & MECHANISM OF ACTION	DOSING GUIDELINES	PHARMACO-KINETICS	ADVERSE EFFECTS	NOTES
Heparin	Anticoagulant; Potentiates the action of antithrombin III, inactivating thrombin and the activation of factors IX, X, XI, XII, and plasmin Prevents conversion of fibrinogen to fibrin	Systemic Heparinization Loading Dose: 75 Units/kg IV over 10 min Maintenance Infusion: < 1yr 28 Units/kg/hr > 1 yr 20 Units/kg/hr	APTT Goal: 60-85 sec Reflects an antifactor Xa level of 0.35-0.7 units/ml (adjust per institutional guidelines). Monitor 4 hrs after loading dose and any change in dose. Once stable, monitor once or twice daily (Use APTT unless levels vary significantly, then consider monitoring by antifactor-Xa levels).	Hemorrhage, development of heparin-induced thrombocytopenia (HIT)	APTT Adjustment < 50 --- Bolus with 50 Unit/kg and increase rate by 10% 50-59 --- Increase rate by 10% 60-85 --- No change 86-95 --- Decrease rate by 10% 96-120 --- Hold for 30 min then decrease rate by 10% > 120 --- Hold for 1 hr then decrease rate by 15%

Hydralazine	Peripheral vasodilator	Pediatrics: 0.1 to 0.2 mg/kg/dose IV (maximum 20 mg) every 4 to 6 hrs Adults: 5-10 mg/dose IV every 4 to 6 hrs (max 40 mg/dose)	$T_{1/2}$ = 2-8 hrs in adults Hepatic metabolism	Tachycardia, flushing, edema, headache, dizziness, rash, emesis, diarrhea, arthralgias, peripheral neuropathy (due to pyridoxine-deficiency), lupus-like syndrome	Available in tablet form; can be prepared as an oral liquid (see references).
Hydrochloro-thiazide	Thiazide diuretic; inhibits Na+ reabsorption in the distal tubule	Pediatrics: 2-4 mg/kg/day PO once daily or divided and given BID Adults: 25-50 mg once daily (max 200 mg/day)	$T_{1/2}$ = 5-15 hrs in adults Excreted unchanged in the urine	Hypotension, electrolyte imbalances, headache, dizziness, weakness, diarrhea, rash, photosensitivity, agranulocytosis, thrombocytopenia	Available in tablet form; no longer commercially available in liquid dosage form.

Common Cardiac Pharmaceuticals

DRUG NAME	CLASS & MECHANISM OF ACTION	DOSING GUIDELINES	PHARMACO-KINETICS	ADVERSE EFFECTS	NOTES
Ibutilide	Class III antiarrhythmic; produces dose-related prolongation of the QT interval; used for rapid conversion of atrial fibrillation or flutter	Pediatrics: 0.01 mg IV infused over 10 min; if no response, dose may be repeated after 10 min Adults (> 60 kg): 1 mg IV infused over 10 min	$T_{1/2}$ = 6 hrs >80% renal excretion; < 10% metabolized to active and inactive compounds	Arrhythmias, hypertension, headache, nausea	Additive effect with other drugs that prolong the QT interval
Isoproterenol	Synthetic catecholamine β_1 agonist	0.05 to 2 mcg/kg/min IV	$T_{1/2}$ = 2-2.5 min Metabolized throughout body	Arrhythmias, hypertension, anxiety, emesis, weakness, tremor	Not compatible with alkaline solutions (e.g. sodium bicarbonate). Tolerance may develop.

390

Common Cardiac Pharmaceuticals

Isradipine	Dihydropyridine calcium channel blocker (reduces SVR with little effect on myocardium)	Pediatrics: 0.1 - 0.5 mg/kg/day PO divided and given QD-TID Adults: 2.5-10 mg PO BID of the immediate release product (max 20 mg/day)	$T_{1/2}$ = 3-8 hrs in adults Hepatic metabolism	Hypotension, edema, headache, dizziness, flushing, tachycardia, weakness, cramps, nausea, rash	Available in tablet form; can be prepared as an oral liquid (see references)
Ketamine	Sedative with mild analgesic properties; produces dissociative amnesia	Pediatrics: 0.5-2 mg/kg/dose IV 3-7 mg/kg/dose IM Adults: 1-2 mg/kg IV	Onset: 1-5 min Duration: 1-2 hrs $T_{1/2}$ = 2.5 hrs Hepatic metabolism	Respiratory depression with rapid bolus, hypertension, arrhythmias, enhanced muscle tone, laryngospasm, hypersalivation **Contraindication:** increased ICP	Administer atropine (0.01 mg/kg) or glycopyrrolate (4-10 mcg/kg IV) before dose to decrease oral secretions.

DRUG NAME	CLASS & MECHANISM OF ACTION	DOSING GUIDELINES	PHARMACOKINETICS	ADVERSE EFFECTS	NOTES
Labetalol	α_1 and non-specific β-adrenergic blocking agent; antihypertensive	Intermittent dose: 0.2 - 1 mg/kg/dose (max 20 mg/dose) Infusion: 0.25 -4 mg/kg/hr	$T_{1/2}$ = 5-8 hrs Extensive first-pass effect; metabolized by hepatic glucuronide conjugation	Hypotension, bradycardia, drowsiness, dizziness, headache, rash, nausea, dry mouth, urinary retention, bronchospasm	
Lidocaine	Class IB antiarrhythmic Suppresses automaticity of ventricles and His-Purkinje system	Loading dose: 1 mg/kg IV (max 100 mg) Infusion: 20-50 mcg/kg/min IV	$T_{1/2}$ = 1-3 hrs Hepatic metabolism to active compounds	Bradycardia, heart block, hypotension, seizures, respiratory depression, anxiety, nausea, phlebitis, blurred vision	

Liothyronine	Exogenous triiodothyronine (T3) Used in post-op low cardiac output states.	Pediatrics: 0.2 - 0.8 mcg/kg/dose IV every 4 - 6 hrs as needed	$T_{1/2}$ = 7 hrs in children; up to 16 hrs in infants	Tachycardia, hypotension	Administer centrally.
Lisinopril	ACE inhibitor	Pediatrics: 0.1-0.4 mg/kg/day PO divided and given QD-TID Adults: 10 mg PO QD, up to 40 mg/day	$T_{1/2}$ = 11-13 hrs in adults Renal excretion	Hypotension, tachycardia, headache, dizziness, rash, angioedema, hyperkalemia, neutropenia, agranulocytosis, hepatic dysfunction (rare)	**Adjust dose in patients with renal dysfunction.** Available in tablet form; can be prepared as an oral liquid (see Prinivil® or Zestril® prescribing information)

Common Cardiac Pharmaceuticals

DRUG NAME	CLASS & MECHANISM OF ACTION	DOSING GUIDELINES	PHARMACOKI-NETICS	ADVERSE EFFECTS	NOTES
Lorazepam	Benzodiaz-epine sedative	Pediatrics: 0.05-0.1 mg/kg IV or PO Adults: 0.5-2 mg IV or PO (max 4 mg)	Onset: 1/2-1 hr Duration: 6-8 hrs $T_{1/2}$ = 6-17 hrs Hepatic metabolism	CNS and respiratory depression, hypoten-sion, arrhythmias, vomiting, dizziness, blurred vision, agitation, muscle weakness	Reversal agent: fluma-zenil 0.01 mg/kg every 60 sec, up to a total of 1 mg (See note #3.)
Lorsartan	Angiotensin II receptor antagonist. Blocks the vasocon-strictor and aldosterone-secreting effects of angiotensin II	Pediatrics: 0.7 mg/kg PO QD; max 1.4 mg/kg Adults: 50 mg PO QD; max 100 mg/day	$T_{1/2}$ = 2 hrs (parent compound), 5 hrs (active me-tabolite). Extensive first pass metabolism; converted in part to active metabolite	Hypotension, muscle cramps, dizziness, hypersensitivity reac-tions, angioedema, hyperkalemia, cough (rare), hepatic dysfunction (rare)	Available in tablet form; can be prepared as an oral liquid (see Cozaar® prescribing information/package insert)

Methadone	Opioid sedative/analgesic	Pediatrics: 0.05-0.2 mg/kg/dose PO, IV every 4-6 hrs for 24-48 hrs, then every 12 hrs	Onset: 30-60 minutes PO; 10-20 minutes IV Duration: 6-8 hrs, increasing to 12-24 hrs with repeated dosing $T_{1/2}$ = 20 hrs in children, 35 hrs in adults after repeated dosing Hepatic metabolism	CNS and respiratory depression, hypotension, bradycardia, emesis, pruritus, urinary retention	Long half-life makes it useful for tapering off long-term opioid use. Reversal agent: naloxone (Narcan®) 5-10 mcg/kg/dose every 2-3 min #2
Metolazone	Diuretic, Inhibits sodium reabsortion in the proximal tubule	Pediatrics: 0.2-0.4 mg/kg/day PO divided and given QD-BID Adults: 5-10 mg PO once daily	$T_{1/2}$ = 6-20 hrs (adults) Excreted unchanged in the urine; some enterohepatic recycling	Hypotension, electrolyte imbalances, headache, dizziness, weakness, bitter taste, emesis, diarrhea, rash, SJS/TEN, photosensitivity, agranulocytosis, thrombocytopenia, tinnitus	Available in tablet form; can be prepared as an oral liquid (see references)

Common Cardiac Pharmaceuticals

DRUG NAME	CLASS & MECHANISM OF ACTION	DOSING GUIDELINES	PHARMACOKINETICS	ADVERSE EFFECTS	NOTES
Metoprolol	β_1-adrenergic blocking agent; antihypertensive and Class II antiarrhythmic	Pediatrics: 0.1-0.5 mg/kg/day PO divided BID; titrated up to 2 mg/kg/day as needed Adults: 50-100 mg/day (max 450 mg/day)	$T_{1/2}$ = 3-10 hrs (prolonged in infants) Metabolized; large first-pass effect	Hypotension, bradycardia, fatigue, headache, dizziness, confusion, depression with long-term use, nausea, bronchoconstriction	Loses β_1 selectivity at higher doses Available in tablet form; can be prepared as an oral liquid (see references)
Mexiletine	Class IB antiarrhythmic	Pediatrics: 1.4-5 mg/kg/dose given PO every 8 hrs Adults: 200 mg PO every 8 hrs, increased as needed (max 1.2 gram/day)	$T_{1/2}$ = 10-14 hrs (adults) Hepatic metabolism via cytochrome P450 1A2	Atrial or ventricular arrhythmias, hypotension, bradycardia, dizziness, confusion, rash, nausea, emesis, hepatitis, tremor, diplopia, tinnitus, rare thrombocytopenia, leukopenia, agranulocytosis	Monitor for drug interactions. Available in capsule form; can be prepared as an oral liquid (see references).

Common Cardiac Pharmaceuticals

Midazolam	Benzodiazepine sedative	Procedural sedation: 0.02-0.1 mg/kg IV 0.1-0.15 mg/kg IM 0.25-0.75 mg/kg PO 0.2-0.4 mg/kg intranasal (repeat as needed) Infusion: 0.05-0.2 mg/kg/hr	Onset: 5-15 min Duration: 1/2-2 hrs $T_{1/2}$ = 2-6 hrs (prolonged in neonates) Hepatic metabolism	CNS and respiratory depression, hypotension, arrhythmias, vomiting, dizziness, blurred vision, agitation, muscle weakness	Reversal agent: flumazenil 0.01 mg/kg every 60 sec, up to a total of 1 mg #3
Milrinone	Phophodiesterase 3 inhibitor Inotrope/vasodilator	Loading dose: 50-75 mcg/kg IV over 15 to 60 min Infusion: 0.25-1 mcg/kg/min	$T_{1/2}$ = 1-3 hrs Eliminated unchanged in urine	Arrhythmias, hypotension, headache, hypokalemia; tremor, thrombocytopenia	**Decrease dose in patients with renal dysfunction.** Incompatible with furosemide.

Common Cardiac Pharmaceuticals

DRUG NAME	CLASS & MECHANISM OF ACTION	DOSING GUIDELINES	PHARMACOKINETICS	ADVERSE EFFECTS	NOTES
Morphine	Opioid sedative/analgesic	Pediatrics: Intermittent dose: 0.1-0.2 mg/kg/dose IV, IM every 2-4 hrs, 0.1-0.5 mg/kg/dose PO every 2-4 hrs Infusion: 0.01-0.04 mg/kg/hr Adults: 2.5-10 mg IV, IM every 2-4 hrs	Onset: 5-60 min Duration: 3-7 hrs $T_{1/2}$ = 5-10 hrs Hepatic metabolism to active and inactive compounds	CNS and respiratory depression, hypotension, bradycardia, nausea, vomiting, pruritus, urinary retention	**If using with a benzodiazepine: decrease dose by 25-50% to avoid respiratory depression.** Reversal agent: naloxone (Narcan®) 5-10 mcg/kg/dose every 2-3 min #2
Nesiritide	B-type naturetic peptide Suppresses renin-angiotensin-aldosterone axis, ↓pre- and afterload, produces diuresis	Loading dose: 1 mcg/kg IV over 2 minutes Infusion: 0.005 to 0.02 mcg/kg/min	$T_{1/2}$ = 18 min (in adults) Eliminated by intracellular lysosomal proteolysis, and renal filtration	Hypotension, worsening cardiac failure, arrhythmias, hypersensitivity reactions, renal dysfunction, headache, emesis	Incompatible with heparin, insulin, ethacrynate sodium, bumetanide, furosemide, enalaprilat, and hydralazine. Dosing information from a small number of case reports.

398

Nicardipine	Dihydropyridine calcium channel blocker; Decreases SVR; effect on arteries > veins	1 to 7 mcg/kg/min IV	$T_{1/2}$ = 2-4 hrs Hepatic metabolism to inactive compounds	Hypotension, tachycardia, arrhythmias, edema, hypokalemia, dizziness, headache	
Nifedipine	Dihydropyridine calcium channel blocker (decreases SVR with little effect on myocardium)	Pediatrics: Immediate release: 0.25 - 0.5 mg/kg every 4 to 6 hrs (max 10 mg single dose) Extended release: 0.25 - 0.9 mg/kg/day PO QD Adults: Extended release 30-60 mg QD	Immediate release: onset 20-30 min, duration 4-8 hrs Extended release: onset 2 hrs, duration 24 hrs $T_{1/2}$ = 2-5 hrs in adults Hepatic metabolism	Hypotension, arrhythmias, edema, headache, nausea, gingival hyperplasia, blood dyscrasias (rare) hepatic dysfunction (rare), diaphoresis	Available in liquid-filled capsules. The capsule contents can be withdrawn and given orally; the concentration of drug in the 10 mg immediate release capsules is approximately 10 mg/0.34 mL. Capsule contents are very light sensitive.

Common Cardiac Pharmaceuticals

DRUG NAME	CLASS & MECHANISM OF ACTION	DOSING GUIDELINES	PHARMACO-KINETICS	ADVERSE EFFECTS	NOTES
Nitric oxide	Pulmonary vasodilator	10-20 ppm delivered as inhaled gas	$T_{1/2}$ = 100-130 ms Inactivated by hemoglobin	Hypotension, inhibition of platelet aggregation, formation of NO_2 and peroxynitrite, methemoglobin-emia	
Nitroglycerin	Coronary and arterial vasodilator; effect on veins>arteries	0.25 to 20 mcg/kg/min IV	$T_{1/2}$ = 1-4 min	Hypotension, flushing, brady-cardia, reflex tachycardia, headache, emesis, diaphoresis	Tolerance develops after 1 to 2 days Use non-PVC tubing Contains propylene glycol, a cardiotoxin

Common Cardiac Pharmaceuticals

Drug	Action	Dose	Metabolism	Adverse Effects	Notes
Nitroprusside	Vasodilator; Decreases SVR by direct effect on vascular smooth muscle; equivalent effect on veins and arteries	0.3-10 mcg/kg/min IV	$T_{1/2}$ < 10 min Converted to cyanide by erythrocyte and tissue sulfhydryl group interactions; converted to thiocyanate by hepatic rhodanase	Hypotension, headache, ↑ICP, emesis, weakness, diaphoresis, Thiocyanate toxicity (in renal dysfunction) or cyanide toxicity (in hepatic dysfunction)	To minimize toxicity, infuse at < 4 mcg/kg/min or for less than 3 days
Norepinephrine	Endogenous catecholamine; β_1 agonist α agonist (predominant effect)	0.05 to 2 mcg/kg/min IV	$T_{1/2}$ = 1-2 min Metabolized by monoamine oxidase and catechol-O-methyltransferase	Arrhythmias, hypertension, emesis, diaphoresis, dyspnea	Administer centrally; extravasation risk. Administer phentolamine as soon as possible following extravasation.

Common Cardiac Pharmaceuticals

DRUG NAME	CLASS & MECHANISM OF ACTION	DOSING GUIDELINES	PHARMACO-KINETICS	ADVERSE EFFECTS	NOTES
Oxycodone	Opioid sedative, analgesic	Pediatrics: 0.05-0.15 mg/kg/dose PO every 4-6 hrs (max 5 mg per dose)	Onset: 10-15 minutes Duration: 4-5 hrs $T_{1/2}$ = 1-3 hrs in children Hepatic metabolism to low concentrations of active metabolites	CNS and respiratory depression, hypotension, bradycardia, emesis, pruritus, urinary retention	Watch for acetaminophen toxicity with repeated doses of combination products Reversal agent: naloxone (Narcan®) 5-10 mcg/kg/dose every 2-3 min #2
Pentobarbital	Barbiturate, sedative	Pediatrics: 1-2 mg/kg/dose IV, IM, PO, PR may be repeated up to a max dose of 100 mg or 6 mg/kg	Onset IV 1 min, IM 10-15 min, PO/PR 15-60 min Duration: 1-4 hrs $T_{1/2}$ = 20-25 hrs Hepatic metabolism	Dose-dependent CNS depression, myocardial depression, hypotension, emesis, laryngospasm, bronchospasm, hypothermia; respiratory depression with rapid administration of large doses	Cannot be used during painful procedures (hyperalgesic). Administer at a rate < 50 mg/min. Injection contains 40% propylene glycol, a cardiotoxin.

Phenylephrine	Synthetic catecholamine α agonist. Weak β_1 agonist	0.1- 0.5 mcg/kg/min IV	$T_{1/2}$ = 2.5 hours. Metabolized by hepatic and intestinal monoamine oxidase	Hypertension, arrhythmias, bradycardia, tremor	Administer centrally; extravasation risk. Administer phentolamine as soon as possible following extravasation.
Prasugrel	Inhibits platelet aggregation through irreversible binding of its active metabolite to the $P2Y_{12}$ ADP receptor on platelets	Adults < 60 kg: 5 mg PO once daily. Adults > 60 kg: 10 mg PO once daily. Pediatric dosing not yet established	$T_{1/2}$ = 2 to 15 hrs in adults. Rapidly hydrolyzed in the intestine to the active form; further metabolized by CYP3A4, 2B6, 2C9, and 2C19	Hemorrhage, thrombotic thrombocytopenic purpura, hypertension, edema, headache, dizziness, rash, GI upset, arthralgias, hypercholesterolemia	Should be administered with aspirin. Available only in tablet form

Common Cardiac Pharmaceuticals

DRUG NAME	CLASS & MECHANISM OF ACTION	DOSING GUIDELINES	PHARMACO-KINETICS	ADVERSE EFFECTS	NOTES
Procainamide	Class IA antiarrhythmic; decreases myocardial excitability and conduction velocity; depresses myocardial contractility	Loading dose: 15 mg/kg IV over 30-60 minutes Infusion: 20-80 mcg/kg/min (max 2 gm/day)	$T_{1/2}$ = 1.7 hrs (procainamide); 6 hrs (N-acetylprocainamide (NAPA) Metabolized in liver to active NAPA	Hypotension, arrhythmias, heart block, QT prolongation, severe blood dyscrasias, lupus-like syndrome, elevated liver enzymes, emesis	Therapeutic serum concentrations: Procainamide: 4 to 10 mcg/mL Sum of procainamide and NAPA: 10 to 30 mcg/mL

| Propafenone | Class IC antiarrhythmic with local anesthetic effects and direct myocardial membrane stabilizing effects | Pediatrics: Initial dose 8-10 mg/kg/day (100-300 mg/m^2/day) divided and given PO BID or TID; increased every 3-4 days as need

Adults: initiate therapy with 150 mg immediate release tablets PO TID, increase every 3-4 days as needed to max 300 mg TID (or 325 mg BID using extended release capsules) | $T_{1/2}$ = 2-10 hrs

Extensive hepatic metabolism via CYP2D6 and CYP3A4 | Arrhythmias, hypotension, dizziness, ataxia, fatigue, headache, lack of appetite, constipation, blurred vision, dyspnea, weakness, dry mouth, rash, increased serum transaminases | Additive effect with other drugs that prolong the QT interval; potential interactions with drugs altering CYP2D6 or 3A4 function

Differences in CYP enzyme phenotypes may result in variations in clinical response and risk for toxicity.

Available in tablet form; can be prepared as an oral liquid (see references) |

Common Cardiac Pharmaceuticals

DRUG NAME	CLASS & MECHANISM OF ACTION	DOSING GUIDELINES	PHARMACO-KINETICS	ADVERSE EFFECTS	NOTES
Propofol	Sedative with mild analgesic properties	Pediatrics: Procedural sedation: 1-3 mg/kg/dose IV, may be repeated Infusion: 50-300 mcg/kg/min	Onset: 30 sec-1 min Duration: 35-10 min $T_{1/2}$ = 1-3 days after repeated administration Hepatic metabolism	Apnea, hypotension, nausea, twitching or movement, burning or stinging at infusion site	Give with lidocaine to reduce pain of injection. Prolonged administration associated with drug accumulation and propofol infusion syndrome (metabolic acidosis, hyperkalemia, lipemia, hepatotoxicity, cardiac and renal failure).
Propranolol	Nonselective β-adrenergic blocking agent; antihypertensive and Class II antiarrhythmic	Pediatrics: Initial: 0.5-1 mg/kg/day PO divided TID/QID; up to 2-4 mg/kg/day; higher doses may be needed for Tet spells (up to 15 mg/kg/day) Adults: 60-80 mg/day PO divided and given TID/QID up to 640 mg/day	$T_{1/2}$ = 4-6 hrs (prolonged with hepatic dysfunction) Hepatic metabolism	Hypotension, bradycardia, fatigue, headache, dizziness, confusion, depression with long-term use, nausea, bronchoconstriction	**NOTE: IV dose (0.01 to 0.1 mg/kg; max 3 mg) is not equivalent to PO dose.** Available as an oral liquid (4 mg/mL and 8 mg/mL).

Sildenafil	Phosphodiesterase 5 inhibitor; pulmonary vasodilator	Pediatrics: 0.25-1 mg/kg/dose PO every 4-8 hrs Adults: 20-60 mg PO TID	$T_{1/2}$ = 4 hrs in adults Hepatic metabolism	Headache, flushing, nausea, diarrhea, rash, vision changes; rare reports in adults of arrhythmias, priapism, migraine, paresthesias, tremor, or hypersensitivity reactions	Available in tablet form; can be prepared as an oral liquid (see references).
Sotalol	Class II/III antiarrhythmic; nonselective β-adrenergic blocking agent	Infants > 2 months: see dosing graph in the product information for Betapace® Children > 2 months: Initial: 30 mg/m2/dose given PO TID or 2 mg/kg/day divided BID/TID; titrate as needed no more frequently than every 3 days; max 180 mg/m2/day or 8 mg/kg/day Adults: Initial 80 mg BID; titrate every 3 days up to 320 mg/day	$T_{1/2}$ = 7-12 hrs Renal elimination as unchanged drug	Arrhythmias, including QT prolongation and torsade de pointes, hypotension, dizziness, anxiety, headache, rash, nausea, vomiting, diarrhea, dyspnea, diaphoresis	Available in tablet form; can be prepared as an oral liquid (see Betapace® prescribing information package insert).

Common Cardiac Pharmaceuticals

DRUG NAME	CLASS & MECHANISM OF ACTION	DOSING GUIDELINES	PHARMACO-KINETICS	ADVERSE EFFECTS	NOTES
Spirono-lactone	Aldosterone antagonist; Increases sodium, chloride, and water excretion in the distal tubule.	Pediatrics: 1-3 mg/kg/day PO given QD or divided and given BID Adults: 25-200 mg/day PO daily or divided and given BID	$T_{1/2}$ = 1-2 hrs in adults Metabolized to active canrenone (T = 13-24 hr)	Electrolyte imbalances (hyperkalemia), arrhythmias, headache, weakness, rash, emesis, diarrhea, dysuria, agranulocytosis, gynecomastia, menstrual changes	**Use with caution in patients receiving potassium supplements while on multiple diuretic therapy.** Available in tablet form; can be prepared as an oral liquid (see references).

Common Cardiac Pharmaceuticals

Tadalafil	Phosphodiesterase 5 inhibitor; pulmonary vasodilator	Adolescents and Adults: 40 mg PO once daily Pediatric dosing not yet established	$T_{1/2}$ = 15 hrs in adults Hepatic metabolism via CPY3A4	Headache, flushing, myalgias, nausea, diarrhea, rash, vision changes, priapism	Available only in tablet form
Treprostinil	Pulmonary vasodilator	Initiate at 2-4 ng/kg/min IV/ subcutaneously and titrate by 1-2 ng/kg/min intervals in new patients; see prescribing information for conversion from epoprostenol to treprostinil	$T_{1/2}$ = 4 hrs Hepatic metabolism	Infusion site reactions, dizziness, headache, chest pain, flushing, jaw pain, anxiety, rash, edema, nausea, diarrhea	Available in a solution for inhalation; pediatric dosing with this product is not yet established

409

Common Cardiac Pharmaceuticals

DRUG NAME	CLASS & MECHANISM OF ACTION	DOSING GUIDELINES	PHARMACO-KINETICS	ADVERSE EFFECTS	NOTES
Valsartan	Angiotensin II receptor antagonist; Blocks the vasoconstrictor and aldosterone-secreting effects of angiotensin II	Children 6-16 yrs: initial dose 1.3 mg/kg PO once daily, increased as needed to max 2.7 mg/kg or 160 mg Adults: initial 80 or 160 mg PO once daily, increase as needed to max 320 mg	$T_{1/2}$ = 6 hrs Primarily excreted as unchanged drug; approximately 20% of dose metabolized to inactive compound	Hypotension, muscle cramps, dizziness, hypersensitivity reactions, angioedema, hyperkalemia, cough (rare), hepatic dysfunction (rare)	Available in tablet form; can be prepared as an oral liquid (see references)
Vasopressin	Endogenous pituitary hormone; Potent vasoconstrictor; increases water permeability in the distal convoluted tubule and collecting duct, decreasing urine volume	Pediatrics: 0.3 - 2 milliunits/kg/min IV Adults: pulseless arrest 40 units IV/IO	$T_{1/2}$ = 10-35 min Metabolized in the liver and kidneys	Myocardial, renal, and/or gut ischemia, venous thrombosis, hypertension, arrhythmias, fluid overload, fever, headache, hyponatremia, nausea, emesis, tremor, bronchospasm, diaphoresis	Administer centrally; extravasation risk.

Common Cardiac Pharmaceuticals

Drug	Mechanism	Dosing	Pharmacokinetics / Monitoring	Adverse Effects	Dose Adjustment
Warfarin	Anticoagulant; Vitamin K antagonist; Interferes with hepatic synthesis of factors II, VII, IX, and X	Initial Dose: 0.2 mg/kg PO given once daily (Day 1 for goal INR of 2-3): • adjust dose as needed for different INR goals Adolescents and Adults: initial dose 2-5 mg PO once daily Overlap with heparin for 3-5 days or until INR therapeutic x 48 hrs.	$T_{1/2}$ = 40 hrs in adults Hepatic metabolism via cytochrome P450 2C9, 2C19, 1A2, and 3A4 Monitoring: INR Goal: Thromboembolic disease, cardiomyopathy, aneurysms from Kawasaki's, atrial fibrillation, post-Fontan, valvular disease, or use of biologic valves: 2-3 Mechanical valves: 2.5-3.5 Low-dose therapy: 1.5-1.9	Hemorrhage, necrosis of the skin early in therapy, edema, headache, GI upset, hematuria, hepatic dysfunction, hypersensitivity reactions	Days 2-4 (based on a goal INR of 2-3) INR — Adjustment 1.1-1.3 — Repeat day 1 dose 1.4-1.9 — 50% of day 1 dose 2-3 — 50% of day 1 dose 3.1-3.5 — 25% of day 1 dose > 3.5 — Hold until < 3.5 Maintenance INR — Adjustment 1.1-1.4 — Increase by 20% 1.5-1.9 — Increase by 10% 2-3 — No change 3.1-3.5 — Decrease by 10% > 3.5 — Hold until < 3.5, then decrease dose by 20%

NOTES AND REFERENCES

Notes:

1. Maximum concentrations for infusion should be used only with central venous access.

2. Naloxone (Narcan) doses listed above are used for partial reversal; for a rapid, full reversal, use 2 mg.

3. Flumazenil has limited efficacy in reversing benzodiazepine-induced respiratory depression due to its short duration of action; provide adequate ventilatory support and repeat as needed.

References:

1. Nahata, M. C., Morosco, R. S., Hipple, T. F. Stability of amiodarone in extemporaneous oral suspensions prepared from commercially available vehicles. *Journal of Pediatric Pharmacy Practice* 1999; 4:186-9.

2. Nahata, M. C., Morosco, R. S., Hipple, T. F. Stability of amlodipine besylate in two liquid dosage forms. *Journal of the American Pharmacists Association* 1999; 39:375-7.

3. Garner, S. S., Wiest, D. B., Reynolds, E. R. Stability of atenolol in an extemporaneously compounded oral liquid. *American Journal of Hospital Pharmacy* 1994; 51:508-11.

4. Nahata, M. C., Morosco, R. S., Hipple, T. F. Stability of captopril in three liquid dosage forms. *American Journal of Hospital Pharmacy* 1994; 51:95-6.

5. Buck, M. L. Use of carvedilol in children with cardiac failure. *Pediatric Pharmacotherapy* 2005; 11(2):1-4. Available at http://www.healthsystem.virginia.edu/internet/pediatrics/education/pharmnews.cfm

6. Levinson, M. L., Johnson, C. E. Stability of an extemporaneously compounded clonidine hydrochloride oral

liquid. *American Journal of Hospital Pharmacy* 1992;
49:122-5.

7. Allen, L. V., Erickson, M. A. Stability of baclofen, captopril, dilitazem hydrochloride, dipyridamole, and flecainide
   acetate in extemporaneously compounded oral liquids.
   American Journal of Health-System Pharmacy 1996;
   53:2179-84.

8. Nahata, M. C., Morosco, R. S., Hipple, T. F. Stability of
   enalapril maleate in three extemporaneously prepared oral
   liquids. *American Journal of Health-System Pharmacy*
   1998; 55:1155-7.

9. Allen, L. V., Erickson, M. A. Stability of labetalol hydrochloride, metoprolol tartrate, verapamil hydrochloride,
   and spironolactone with hydrochlorothiazide in extemporaneously compounded oral liquids. *American Journal of
   Health-System Pharmacy* 1996; 53:2304-9.

10. Wiest, D. B., Garner, S. S., Pagacz, L. R. Stability of
    flecainide acetate in an extemporaneously compounded
    oral suspension. *American Journal of Hospital Pharmacy*
    1992; 49:1467-70.

11. Allen, L. V., Erickson, M. A. Stability of alprazolam,
    chloroquine phosphate, cisapride, enalapril maleate, and
    hydralazine hydrochloride in extemporaneously com-
    pounded oral liquids. *American Journal of Health-System
    Pharmacy* 1998; 55:1915-20.

12. MacDonald, J. L., Johnson, C. E., Jacobson, P. Stability
    of isradipine in an extemporaneously compounded oral
    liquid. *American Journal of Hospital Pharmacy* 1994;
    51:2409-11.

13. Allen, L. V., Erickson, M. A. Stability of ketoconazole,
    metolazone, metronidazole, procainamide hydrochloride,
    and spironolactone in extemporaneously compounded oral
    liquids. *American Journal of Health-System Pharmacy*
    1996; 53:2073-8.

14. Nahata, M. C., Morosco, R. S., Hipple, T. S. Stability
    of mexiletine in two extemporaneous liquid formula-

413

tions stored under refrigeration and at room temperature. *Journal of the American Pharmacists Association* 2000; 40:257-9.

15. Nahata, M. C., Morosco, R. S., Brady, M. T. Extemporaneous sildenafil citrate oral suspensions for the treatment of pulmonary hypertension in children. *American Journal of Health-System Pharmacy* 2006; 63:254-7.

16. Barnes, S., Shields, B., Bonney, W., et al. The pediatric cardiology pharmacopoeia: 2004 update. *Pediatric Cardiology* 2004; 25:623-646.

17. Monagle, P., Chalmers, E., Chan, A., et al. Antithrombotic therapy in neonates and children: American College of Chest Physicians Evidence-based Clinical Practice Guidelines (8th edition). *CHEST* 2008; 133:887-968.

18. Taketomo, C.K., Hodding, J. H., Kraus, D.M. **Pediatric Dosage Handbook**. 16th ed. Hudson, Ohio: Lexi-Comp, Inc., 2009.

INDEX